# Nutritional Lithium: A Cinderella Story

# Nutritional Lithium:
# A Cinderella Story

### The Untold Tale of a Mineral That Transforms Lives and Heals the Brain

James M. Greenblatt MD & Kayla Grossmann RN

Copyright © 2016 James M. Greenblatt MD & Kayla Grossmann RN
All rights reserved.

ISBN: 1511716487
ISBN 13: 9781511716482
Library of Congress Control Number: 2016901247
CreateSpace Independent Publishing Platform
North Charleston, South Carolina

# Disclaimer

The information presented in this book has not been evaluated or approved by the U.S. Food and Drug Administration. The products discussed in this book are not intended to diagnose, treat, cure or prevent any disease.

This book is designed to provide information on the current available research on low dose lithium. This book is not intended, nor should it be used, as a substitute for the medical advice of physicians. The reader should regularly consult a physician in matters relating to his/her health and particularly with respect to any symptoms that may require diagnosis or medical attention. Nutritional supplements should be taken under the supervision of a health care professional.

Additionally, some names and identifying details have been changed to protect the privacy of individuals.

# Contents

| | | |
|---|---|---|
| Foreword | Misunderstood Mineral | ix |
| Introduction | The Besieged Brain: The Increased Rates in Neurological and Psychiatric Illnesses | xv |
| Chapter 1 | Nutritional Psychiatry: The Future is Now | 1 |
| Chapter 2 | From Prescription Pad to Health Food Store | 7 |
| Chapter 3 | The History of Lithium: How A Mineral Becomes A Medicine | 15 |
| Chapter 4 | Nutritional Lithium as a Dietary Supplement | 23 |
| Chapter 5 | Lithium as a Mineral: Neuroprotection and Brain Health | 39 |
| Chapter 6 | Lithium as a Mineral: Orchestrating Our Genes | 61 |
| Chapter 7 | Lithium as a Medicine: Dementia & Alzheimer's Disease | 72 |
| Chapter 8 | Lithium as a Medicine: Parkinson's Disease | 87 |
| Chapter 9 | Lithium as a Medicine: Mood Disorders | 103 |
| Chapter 10 | Lithium as a Medicine: Suicide Prevention | 124 |
| Chapter 11 | Lithium as a Medicine: Irritability, Anger and Aggression | 138 |
| Chapter 12 | Lithium as a Medicine: Addiction and Substance Abuse | 153 |
| Chapter 13 | Lithium as a Medicine: Eating Disorders and Attention-Deficit Hyperactivity Disorder | 168 |
| Chapter 14 | Lithium as a Medicine: Lyme Disease, Headaches, Glaucoma, and Fibromyalgia | 176 |

| | | |
|---|---|---|
| Chapter 15 | The Role of Lithium in Integrative Psychiatry | 188 |
| | Author Bios | 197 |
| | Appendix | 199 |
| | Resources | 205 |

# Foreword

## MISUNDERSTOOD MINERAL
Jonathan Wright MD, ND (hon)

Sometime in the late 1970s or early 1980s, a 21 year old woman came to see me at Tahoma Clinic. She'd been in a few times before as a teenager for relatively minor health problems; her parents had been in several times about issues that mostly traced back to the alcoholism they'd both suffered from since they were young (except when her mother was pregnant with her, she had been told).

She told me she wasn't ill, but wanted to know if it would be alright for her to take the same amount of lithium her parents were each taking, once daily. However, she had told me at a prior visit that she had "never swallowed as much as one drop of alcohol in my whole lifetime", motivated by what she'd seen it do to her parents themselves and to their marriage.

At that visit she'd also told me that her parents had been doing much better—although not perfectly—since starting on daily lithium. Her father wasn't losing his temper as much, not yelling nearly as much, and was definitely less irritable. Her mother was even happy some of the time now, not depressed and weepy all the time as she'd been before. And no, they hadn't stopped drinking alcohol, but the amount and frequency had both diminished significantly.

# Foreword

So why did she want to take lithium herself? Had she started drinking alcohol since her last visit? No, she quietly assured me, she hadn't, and never would. So, why? Before answering, she sat upright in her chair, stared at me, and then asked: "Don't I have the same genetics as my parents?" She was of course correct; couldn't argue with that!

She continued to say that she'd observed her parents feeling better and getting along better since shortly after starting the lithium, and although her own behavior wasn't—and never would be, she repeated—influenced by personal alcohol use, she thought she might feel better too if she took the same amount of lithium they did every day. Her parents had advised her to check with me, and so here she was.

We reviewed lithium safety first. Even though adverse effects were very unlikely if she used the same quantities her parents were using, why not do something that might significantly lower if not eliminate any chance of lithium causing her problems? She agreed that prevention was probably better than cure, and asked what that might be.

Dr. David Horrobin had taught us at a seminar that essential fatty acids would eliminate or reduce lithium toxicity. Although Dr. Horrobin and his colleague Dr. Lieb had used safflower oil in a preliminary study, after studying essential fatty acids it appeared to me that flaxseed oil would be a better choice.

At different times in the years after Dr. Horrobin's seminar, two severely bipolar individuals were referred to me by a psychiatrist who'd helped them keep their severe bipolar symptoms under control for several years with high dose lithium. Then each had signs and symptoms of lithium toxicity appear, including tremor, nausea, rising blood pressure. Excess protein was found in their urine.

But even a small reduction in lithium dose caused their bipolar symptoms to flare, so each wanted to stay with the higher doses of lithium. The psychiatrist referred them to me. Each was advised to take flaxseed oil, one tablespoonful thrice daily (along with vitamin E 400 IU twice daily), and for both individuals the lithium toxicity slowly went away in three to four weeks.

For her, large quantities of flaxseed oil itself were very likely not needed, and there was an alternative means of getting the same oil that many had told me was even tasty, ground flaxseed itself, two level tablespoonfuls daily. She agreed it would be easy to stir that into the oatmeal she liked to eat for breakfast

In succeeding years—it wasn't known at that time—researchers have found that ground flaxseed also reduces risk of breast cancer, improves progesterone-to-estrogen ratios (which often lessens PMS), increases the percentage of ovulatory cycles, and even raises a woman's testosterone levels slightly. But enough about ground flaxseed, back to lithium…..

She didn't return for nearly a year. There was definitely a change in her personality; she seemed more confident, and didn't wait to be asked about what she had in mind for the visit. When we were done with that concern, she said she had something to tell me about herself that she hadn't mentioned at any prior visit.

"I never had any close friends when I was growing up" she said. "I thought it was because of my parents; before they started lithium, I didn't want to be around them much either. But even after that, still no close friends. There were very few invitations to parties or to join clubs, and when all the other girls were old enough to have boyfriends, I didn't until I was nineteen, and that lasted less than a month."

"But since I started the lithium and (she smiled) ground flaxseed everyone who knew me in high school says I'm not the same person. A few of the more outspoken ones asked me if I'd been having psychological counseling. I tell them no, I just made a decision about my life and let's leave it at that. I've been invited to more parties in the last few months than in my entire time in high school."

"I've decided to go to college, and I've gotten a job to earn money for it. I've met lots of people at the job, and one of them has been my boyfriend for six and a half months now! Now I understand what the other girls were talking about in the locker room in high school gym. My parents are amazed at the change that's happened to me, so I tell them it's all their fault for taking the lithium you suggested…..the other reason I'm here is to thank you for doing that." Which was very kind of her…

Only a few who use low dose lithium have as dramatic a personality change. Even while keeping close track of lithium research since the 1970s,

# Foreword

it never occurred to me that lithium might be of use for me, personally, until reading a research report published in the year 2000 in *The Lancet*, a British medical journal considered to be among the top few in the world. This report told us that after just four weeks of use of lithium by ten bipolar patients, before and after MRI brain scans showed a significant increase in "grey-matter volume" in eight of the ten!

"Grey matter" is the same as Hercule Poirot's "little grey cells", the brain cells with which we do our thinking! In my time in medical school—which our children say was in the Dark Ages—we'd been told that we have all the brain cells we're going to have by the time we became adult, and after that, it was all downhill for brain cells. One professor told us that we could always tell a skull X-ray from a ninety-year-old, as "the brain is always shrunken".

The median increase in grey cell volume reported in *The Lancet* article was 3% or 24 cubic centimeters, which my computer tells me is the same as 1.46 cubic inches. That's literally billions of new brain cells! As we all can use all the brain cells we can get, and the natural food store had low dose lithium even in the year 2000, it's been on my personal health-maintenance list ever since!

For me, it's not for any mental disorder—although *los federales* at the FDA and the State Medical Board might disagree—but for a continuing supply of new brain cells as the older ones wear out, and as Dr. Greenblatt and Kayla Grossmann tell us so well in this book, to support, protect and improve my overall brain health. Possibly most importantly, lithium—along with testosterone for men, estrogen for women, and curcumin (the major component of the spice turmeric)—very significantly cuts Alzheimer's risk for all of us!

And low dose lithium for brain health and other aspects of health is not all you'll read in this book! Just one example, as this foreword is getting long: Chapter 1 ("Nutritional Psychiatry") is relevant to all of medicine, not just psychiatry. As human bodies have been made from the natural substances and natural energies of planet Earth, without any patent medicines—also called "pharmaceuticals" or "drugs"—in the original design, it's obvious that to improve and maintain the health of our bodies we should use those same natural substances and energies!

What would you say if a mechanic tried to convince that the best way to fix your Honda is with Ford parts? You'd probably listen and then take your

# Nutritional Lithium: A Cinderella Story

car for repairs with Honda parts! So why trust your health, especially long-term intake of substances not only never before found in human bodies, but never before found on planet Earth?

Certainly there are occasional emergencies when a patent medicine can be lifesaving, but when the emergency is over, for the best of health for the rest of our lives it's always best to return to those natural substances and energies which have kept human bodies healthy for 99.99% of the time humanity has been on planet Earth. As important as it is—and after reading this book, you'll be more than convinced—low dose lithium is but one of many, many substances found on planet Earth that will help us improve and maintain health.

If you haven't done so already, please find and work with a physician skilled and knowledgeable in natural medicine! In addition to using substances and energies that really have a place and function in your body, physicians using natural substances and energies *always look for the cause of health problems first, and treat the cause!* Patent medicines ("pharmaceuticals", drugs) can't possibly treat the cause of any illness since the cause is never, ever a lack of patent medicines!

And even when the cause can't be found, you'll find that properly used natural substances and energies are more effective at controlling and improving health problems than patent medicines, and with many, many, many fewer adverse effects.

To find such a physician, refer to the Resources section toward the end of this book. Thanks very much to Dr. Greenblatt and Kayla Grossmann for researching and writing it, and may it help you to be well!

Jonathan V. Wright MD, ND (hon)<br>
Tahoma Clinic<br>
Tukwila, Washington<br>
www.tahomaclinic.com

References

Lieb, J. & Horrobin, D. F. (1981). Treatment of lithium-induced tremor and familial essential tremor with essential fatty acids. *Progress In Lipid Research, 20,* 535-7.

Moore, G. J., Bebchuk, J. M., Wilds, I. B., Chen, G., & Menji, H. K. (2000). Lithium-induced increase in human brain grey matter. *Lancet, 356*(9237), 1241-1242.

# Introduction

## The Besieged Brain: The Increased Rates of Neurological and Psychiatric Illnesses

Chronic diseases like cancer, heart disease, and diabetes compromise quality of life for millions of Americans. Yet as tragic a burden as these diseases are, none of them is the greatest cause of disability among Americans. Surprisingly to many, mental disorders have become the leading cause of disability nationwide. In our culture, characterized by a stressful and hurried lifestyle and increasing exposure to environmental pollution, our brains are besieged by more adversity and challenge than ever before.

The scientific community has published unquestionable data and evidence that rates of mental illness are on the rise. A large survey of randomly selected adults found that a staggering 46% of Americans have had at least one mental illness within four basic types at some time during their lives (Angell, 2011). These types are anxiety disorders, including phobias and post-traumatic stress disorder (PTSD); mood disorders, including major depression and bipolar disorder; impulse disorders, most commonly attention deficit- hyperactivity disorder (ADHD); and substance abuse disorders such as alcoholism and drug abuse. Between 13% and 20% of children living in the U.S. experience a mental disorder in a given year, and surveillance shows that this prevalence is increasing (Perou, et al., 2013). The Centers for Disease Control and Prevention

## Introduction

(CDC, 2013) reported that the suicide rate among Americans aged 35 to 64 increased more than 28% between 1999 and 2010.

Bipolar disorder is also on the increase. The estimated annual number of office visits by youth with a diagnosis of bipolar disorder increased between 1995 and 2003, from 25 visits to 1,003 visits per 100,000. Office visits by adults increased from 905 to 1,679 per 100,000 during the same period. The proportion of young people in a large database of privately insured patients who received outpatient treatment for bipolar disorder increased by 67%, while the proportion who received inpatient treatment increased by 74% (Moreno et al., 2007).

Physicians are also seeing ADHD in much larger numbers of children, brought in by their parents and often referred by the school system. A 2010 U.S. government survey reported that one in ten American children has ADHD—an increase of 22% in just seven years (Visser et al., 2010).

Not only are numbers of diagnoses for mental and emotional disorders going up; the rates of disability for mental illness have also skyrocketed. Since 1955, Americans disabled by mental illness have increased nearly six fold (Whitaker, 2011). The number of people who are disabled by mental disorders and qualify for Supplemental Security Income or Social Security Disability Insurance increased nearly two and a half times between 1987 and 2007, from one in 184 Americans to one in 76. In children the increase is even more astonishing. Mental illness is now the leading cause of disability in children, surpassing physical disabilities including Down syndrome and cerebral palsy. Mental health disability has increased in children by 35 times within just two decades (Angell, 2011).

Rates of neurodegenerative and neurological disorders are also steadily rising. While total mortality fell substantially in the 30-year period between 1980 and 2010, deaths from neurological causes rose significantly in Australia, Canada, Germany, Italy, Spain, the U.K., and the U.S. (Pritchard et al., 2013). Between 2000 and 2010, Alzheimer's disease went from the 25th to the 12th most burdensome disease overall, and from 32nd to 9th in terms of lost years of life. As baby boomers continue aging, 7.1 million people aged 65 and older are expected to have Alzheimer's disease by 2025, a 40% increase from the rate today

(Alzheimer's Association, 2015). Parkinson's disease too is on the rise. Studying 15 countries, researchers estimated that the number of individuals over 50 with Parkinson's is between 4.1 million and 4.6 million. That number is projected to double by 2030, to between 8.7 and 9.3 million (Dorsey et al., 2007).

Perhaps even more astonishing is the increase in psychiatric and neurological disorders that have occurred despite the introduction and wide use during the past four decades of prescription medications to treat these disorders. Despite these discouraging results, the medical model that guides psychiatric thinking is mired in the same old approaches. Operating from the theory that mental disorders are caused by chemical imbalance, most psychiatrists offer only pharmacological treatment. The numbers of prescriptions for psychotropic drugs have increased exponentially (Carlat, 2011). Prescriptions for antidepressants have increased during the last two decades by 400% (National Center for Health Statistics, 2011). It is both concerning and tragic that a larger percentage of the population than ever before report being depressed. Why has the number of patients on disability more than tripled during the past two decades, a period during which many new medicines were introduced, some trumpeted as the next "wonder drug"? And why has the number of children on disability from mental illness skyrocketed from about 16,000 to 600,000? (Whitaker, 2011).

Studies reveal that only about 15% of depressed people treated with medicine stay healthy over the long run; the remaining 85% struggle with chronic depression. During the past several decades, most patients on medications have shifted from experiencing isolated episodes of depression, often years apart, to suffering long-term emotional disability. These long-term effects often go unrecognized, because most studies are short-term, typically lasting only 6 to 8 weeks, at which endpoint the conclusion is reached that antidepressant, anti-anxiety, or anti-psychotic medications work. Robert Whitaker has written extensively about the possibility that psychotropic drugs are effective in the short term, but may exacerbate the chronicity of depression (Whitaker, 2011).

While many psychotropic medications are considered safe, medications can also cause adverse reactions that include weight gain, sexual dysfunction,

## Introduction

sedation, suicidal ideation, and physical symptoms including headache, nausea, and gastrointestinal distress. One study reported that about 40% of patients taking an antidepressant medication experienced side effects, and about 25% of these patients described their side effects as negatively affecting their quality of life (Kirsch, 2011). Visits to emergency rooms due to adverse medication reactions also increased by more than 400% from 2005 to 2011 (SAMHSA, 2013). It is common for physicians to add medications to minimize side effects brought on by existing medications, causing patients to become more vulnerable to developing more side effects. Frustrated, patients may stop taking medications without notifying their doctor and continue to suffer from symptoms.

The human brain comprises the largest percent of total body weight of the brains in all animal species and demands a greater proportion of the body's energy. At rest, the human brain consumes 25% of the body's total available energy, more than double the rate in most other animals (Sherwood et al., 2011). Marine mammals, including whales and dolphins, are the only other species with brains that come close in size and scale. From an evolutionary perspective, these shared features make sense: humans and marine mammals are exceptionally smart. We share incredible gifts—our abilities to learn, remember, communicate, and form complex social groups. The brain, as the master commander of all these processes, needs enough size and power to support these critical functions.

Ironically, some of the physiological traits that predispose us to such an advanced level of cognitive performance also make the brain highly susceptible to damage. The brain depends for fuel on a continuous supply of compounds like oxygen and glucose. Every second of every day these compounds are being transformed through complicated metabolic steps into a usable form of energy. Eventually, this pace takes a toll on the cells. Researchers are now finding that, unlike brain cells in other animals, human brain cells show distinct signs of wear and tear over time. In particular, the mitochondria, or energy storehouses of the cells, start to decrease in efficiency and break down. Signs of oxidative stress, or cellular damage caused by the build-up of metabolic byproducts, also commonly appear in the brains of older adults.

## Nutritional Lithium: A Cinderella Story

The physical structure of the brain also enhances its vulnerability. In order to insulate and protect the neurons, for example, the brain naturally contains a high level of fat in the form of cholesterol and unsaturated essential fatty acids. For the most part, these fats support and nourish the cells. They are present in the neuron cell membranes or the outer covering that serves as the barrier between the cell contents and its surrounding environment. Fatty acids also appear in myelin, an additional insulating coating that wraps around nervous system cells to help electrical signals transmit quickly and efficiently between them.

While the fatty acids in the brain are critical for enhancing structure and communication, they also attract toxins. Many toxic environmental chemicals are fat-soluble, which means they readily accumulate in fatty tissues. Even more damaging, the distinctive chemical structure of unsaturated fatty acids makes them naturally fragile and reactive. A brief exposure to a chemical or abrupt physical force can cause unsaturated fatty acids to rapidly deform or break down, resulting in damage to the cell.

The medical model has achieved only modest benefits in addressing the global burden of brain disorders. Recognizing the tremendous burden of neurological and psychiatric disease on the lives of Americans, President Obama called on the American scientific research community to seek breakthroughs in understanding and treating brain disorders. The initiative, called BRAIN (Brain Research through Advancing Innovative Neurotechnologies), brings together specialists from neuroscience, imaging, and engineering to better understand how thoughts and emotions are registered in the brain.

The brain is an amazing, complicated but vulnerable organ. The intricate processes that are critical for maintaining brain health can be eroded by the wear and tear of stress, aging, inactivity, and exposure to environmental toxins. Psychiatric medications, by altering neurotransmitter levels for short-term gain, may disrupt neuronal pathways and lead to negative long-term outcomes (Whitaker, 2011).

This book is about the often neglected aspect of medicine that offers proven, efficacious interventions to combat the rise of psychiatric illness: nutritional biochemistry. Vitamins and minerals are critical for optimal function of

# Introduction

the human body and are responsible for several basic roles including enzyme activity and protein synthesis. Insufficient vitamin and mineral reserves promote disease states that result in poor brain development, cognitive deficits, and psychiatric symptoms. Lithium, a natural element that is capable of stimulating neuronal growth and repair of damaged neurons, can help mitigate several psychiatric symptoms. Understanding the benefits of low dose lithium can help redefine the treatment and prevention for major psychiatric illnesses.

The field of nutritional psychiatry is based on the conviction that identifying and correcting nutritional deficiencies in the body is the path to restoring the health and optimal function of the molecular magic that supports every facet of our brain health.

# Nutritional Lithium: A Cinderella Story

## INTRODUCTION | References

Alzheimer's Association. (2015). Alzheimer's disease facts and figures. *Alzheimer's & Dementia: The Journal of the Alzheimer's Association, 11*(3), 332.

Angell, M. (2011). The epidemic of mental illness: why? *The New York Review of Books, 58*(11), 2.

Carlat, D. J. (2010). Unhinged: *The trouble with psychiatry—A doctor's revelations about a profession in crisis.* New York, NY, US: Free Press.

Centers for Disease Control and Prevention. (2013). Suicide among adults aged 35-64 years--United States, 1999-2010. *MMWR. Morbidity and Mortality Weekly Report, 62*(17), 321-325.

Dorsey, E. R., Constantinescu, R., Thompson, J. P., Biglan, K. M., Holloway, R. G., Kieburtz, K., & ... Tanner, C. M. (2007). Projected number of people with Parkinson's disease in the most populous nations, 2005 through 2030. *Neurology, 68*(5), 384-386.

Kirsch, I. (2010). *The emperor's new drugs: Exploding the antidepressant myth.* New York, NY, US: Basic Books.

Moreno, C., Laje, G., Blanco, C., Jiang, H., Schmidt, A. B., & Olfson, M. (2007). National trends in the outpatient diagnosis and treatment of bipolar disorder in youth. *Archives of General Psychiatry, 64*(9), 1032-9.

National Center for Health Statistics. (2011). Health, United States, 2010: With special feature on death and dying. Table 95. Hyattsville, MD.

Perou, R., Bitsko, R. H., Blumberg, S. J., Pastor, P., Ghandour, R. M., Gfroerer, J. C., & ... Huang, L. N. (2013). Mental health surveillance among children--United States, 2005-2011. *Morbidity and Mortality Weekly Report. Surveillance Summaries (Washington, D.C.: 2002), 62*(Suppl 2), 1-35.

Pritchard, C., Mayers, A., Baldwin, D. (2013). Changing patterns of neurological mortality in the ten major developed countries—1979-2010. *Public Health 127*(4), 357-68.

Sherwood, C. C., Gordon, A. D., Allen, J. S., Phillips, K. A., Erwin, J. M., Hof, P. R., & Hopkins, W. D. (2011). Aging of the cerebral cortex differs between humans and chimpanzees. *Proceedings of the National Academy of Sciences of the United States of America, 108*(32), 13029- 13034.

# Introduction

Substance Abuse and Mental Health Services Administration (SAMHSA). (2013). *The DAWN Report: Emergency Department Visits Involving Phencyclidine (PCP)*. Rockville, MD: Center for Behavioral Health Statistics and Quality.

Visser, S., Bitsko, R., Danielson, M., Perou, R., & Blumberg, S. (2010). Increasing prevalence of parent-reported attention-deficit/hyperactivity disorder among children--United States, 2003 and 2007. *Morbidity and Mortality Weekly Report, 59*(44), 1439-1443.

Whitaker, R. (2011). *Anatomy of an epidemic: Magic bullets, psychiatric drugs, and the astonishing rise of mental illness in America*. New York, NY, US: Crown Publishers/Random House.

# One

## Nutritional Psychiatry: The Future is Now

We are in the midst of a scientific revolution in understanding brain health. The research that has fueled dramatic developments in our understanding of neuroscience is finally affecting the clinical practice of medicine.

The last major transformation in psychiatry occurred about six decades ago, when imbalances in neurotransmitters, especially serotonin, were identified as factors involved in mental illness. Pharmacology was heralded as the way to cure mental disorders by adjusting chemical imbalances. The pharmacological model has achieved some success in treating mental illness, yet ongoing research has repeatedly demonstrated the clinical contribution of this model is limited. Neurobiological findings during the intervening decades show that pharmacological interventions do not address all aspects of brain metabolism. A positive response from treatment with psychiatric medication is seen about 50%-60% of the time, with these response rates plummeting as patients fail the first round of treatments. Remission occurs only about 30% of the time (Trivedi et al., 2006). Unsurprisingly, then, many people who suffer from mental health disorders receive one prescription after another.

The ten minute "med check" is the norm and established treatment model in psychiatry. The hospital door becomes a revolving door. It is not unusual for outpatients to have sought help from a long parade of medical professionals without achieving freedom from disturbing psychiatric symptoms.

# Nutritional Psychiatry: The Future is Now

A new dramatic shift in neuroscience research illuminates the contribution of nutrition to brain health. Compelling evidence now identifies malnutrition as a critical factor in mental disorders. Accumulating research results show just how nutrition affects brain health. The brain functions at a high metabolic rate and uses a substantial portion of total nutrient intake. It relies on amino acids, fats, vitamins, minerals, and trace elements. These affect both brain structure and function. Diet also influences the function of the immune system, linked closely with mood. The antioxidant defense system relies on the support of nutrients to moderate inflammation and toxins. Nutrition also contributes to neuron plasticity and repair, key functions of mental health. In fact, diet is as critical to psychiatry as it is to cardiology to gastroenterology. Scientific research is accumulating on the nutritional influences of every aspect of health and chronic disease (Kaplan et al., 2015).

The mounting epidemiologic evidence that links nutrition and mental health suggests that correcting nutritional deficiencies could lower rates of psychiatric disorders at both an individual and a population level. Most importantly, nutrition is a critical *modifiable* intervention for preventing and treating psychiatric problems. Unlike a genetic legacy, family background, or life experience, nutritional status is a risk factor for mental illness that can easily be changed.

For psychiatrists to treat mental illnesses as exclusively psychological disorders fails to account for the brain's physiological response to a shortage of essential nutrients. This response occurs regardless of culture, psychological traits, or family pressures. The malnourished brain must be restored with the nutrients it lacks. Just as problematic is treatment of psychological disorders as exclusively biological problems that can be treated simply by medications or adding vitamins.

Viewing mental disorders as exclusively psychological or biological disorders reduces the scope of possible interventions and treatments. Even today, despite advances in public education, people with mental illness suffer not only from their disorder; they also live in the shadows of guilt and self-blame. Stigma still shrouds mental illness partly because of our culture's tendency to explain mental illness in vague psychological terms or simple biological observations treatable with a pill.

A disconnect now exists between results from recent scientific research on mental illness and the treatment models we use. Medical professionals are slow to recognize the contribution of nutrition in disease progression and health. In part, this is because physicians are not trained in nutrition. Medical students do not receive the training they need either to understand the importance of nutrition or how to counsel patients.

Moreover, nutrition does not command attention in the medical community. Pharmaceutical companies invest billions of dollars in research, hoping to create the next blockbuster medication. Nutritional substances, by contrast, are inexpensive and non-patentable. Nutritional medicine has historically been considered "alternative." Holding on to this outdated view, psychiatrists and other mental health professionals have continued to lag behind the rest of medicine in incorporating nutritional therapies into treatment.

The last ten years of scientific research have firmly established that nutritional medicine is no longer considered "alternative" medicine. We now know that what we eat is the foundation of optimal health and a robust brain. A healthy brain leads to a mind that defines our uniqueness, and our uniqueness creates our psychological freedom. This is the foundation of nutritional psychiatry.

Nutrients support the biochemical reactions necessary for optimal brain function. Although nutritional psychiatry is a relatively new discipline, the connection between nutrition and mental health has been recognized for a long time. A classic example involves the story of pellagra, a vitamin B3 deficiency that was common in this country in the early 1900s. Pellagra got its name in 1771 from the Italian phrase for "rough skin." However, the affliction tormented individuals and populations for centuries before it was formally named at the end of the eighteenth century (Rajakumar, 2000). A number of Biblical scholars suggest that some of the torments that afflicted Job were probably symptoms of pellagra.

Patients with pellagra were plagued with skin lesions, intestinal distress, lethargy, and depression. A common finding in pellagra was delusions that are indistinguishable from what we now call schizophrenia. The American medical establishment first focused attention on the problem in the earliest days of the twentieth century, when the disease reached epidemic proportions across the South. For decades doctors were perplexed. In 1915, Joseph Goldberger, a physician in the U.S. Public Health Service, discovered the cause of pellagra that had baffled everyone else. Most investigators had assumed it resulted from something its sufferers ate, most likely corn. Goldberger recognized that it resulted from something they *didn't* eat. He encouraged physicians and the public in areas where pellagra was prevalent to change their diet to include fresh milk, meat, and eggs (Rajakumar, 2000). Goldberger saw that people who ate a more varied diet did not suffer from pellagra. But what he did not fully understand was that the South was effectively suffering a famine of a crucial brain nutrient. Patients who were psychiatrically impaired were deficient in a single nutrient that resulted in devastating and profound effects on brain function even when they consumed sufficient calories.

During the height of pellagra in the South, patients with pellagra occupied up to 50% of all mental health institutions until they succumbed to the disease (Rajakumar, 2000). The accompanying disorientation and psychosis observed in pellagrins led to mistaken diagnoses of schizophrenia. Pellagrins exhibited psychiatric symptoms such as disordered logic, confusion, irritability, agitation, and dementia, particularly in the later stages of the disease. Ultimately, nicotinic acid or vitamin B3 deficiency was identified as the cause of pellagra. Niacin deficiency influences the synthesis of serotonin, causing dysfunctional neural transmission. This mechanism explains the neurological and psychiatric symptoms seen in those suffering from pellagra (Wang & Liang, 2012). More than 30 years after Goldberger identified the cause, pellagra was essentially eliminated as Vitamin B3 was quickly incorporated into American diets. From pellagra we learned that a single nutritional deficiency can manifest with disabling psychiatric symptoms.

Malnutrition has profound effects on mood. Research has consistently shown that a Western diet high in processed foods and low in fruits and vegetables is associated with increased rates of anxiety and depression. A prospective cohort study of 9,000 college graduates in Spain found that those with the highest consumption of fast food had a 40% higher risk of depression. A direct association was also found between commercial baked good consumption and depression. In contrast, a healthy dietary pattern, such as the Mediterranean diet, has been related to a lower risk of depression (Sánchez-Villegas et al., 2012).

Researchers in Australia found a positive correlation between the amount of low-nutrient food products (e.g., processed foods, refined grains, sugary products, beer) consumed and women's mood and anxiety symptoms. The association between diet and mood may be related to inflammation. Western diets are associated with higher levels of C-reactive protein, a marker of low-grade inflammation. Inflammatory processes are also thought to play a role in the onset and maintenance of depressive disorders (Jacka et al., 2010).

Recent scientific findings show that many nutritional elements are important to brain fitness. Nutrients serve as cofactors in almost every enzymatic reaction in the brain. When there are insufficient nutrients, metabolic pathways, including synthesis of neurotransmitters, cannot function at optimum levels. Medications can increase the availability of neurotransmitters, but nutrients naturally supply cofactors to enzymes to optimize the pathways involved in neurotransmitter synthesis.

This book will focus on a single nutrient, lithium, which has far reaching implications for psychological health. Lithium has unique properties capable of relieving psychiatric and neurological symptoms and promoting the health of the brain through the life span.

Not unlike the vitamin B3 deficiency seen in pellagra, lithium deficiency might be responsible for less dramatic, but more insidious, assaults on our psychological well-being including depression, anxiety, dementia, and the unfathomable tragedy of suicide.

## CHAPTER 1 | References

Jacka, F., Pasco, J., Mykletun, A., Williams, L., Hodge, A., O'Reilly, S., & Berk, M. (2010). Association of Western and traditional diets with depression and anxiety in women. *American Journal of Psychiatry, 167*(3), 305-311.

Kaplan, B.J., Rucklidge, J.J., Romijn, A., & McLeod, K. (2015). The emerging field of nutritional mental health: inflammation, the microbiome, oxidative stress, and mitochondrial function. *Clinical Psychological Science, 3*(6), 964-980.

Rajakumar, K. (2000). Pellagra in the United States: a historical perspective. *Southern Medical Journal, 93*(3), 272-277.

Sánchez-Villegas, A., Toledo, E., de Irala, J., Ruiz-Canela, M., Pla-Vidal, J., & Martínez-González, M. (2012). Fast-food and commercial baked goods consumption and the risk of depression. *Public Health Nutrition, 15*(3), 424-432.

Trivedi, M. H., Rush, A. J., Wisniewski, S. R., Nierenberg, A. A., Warden, D., Ritz, L., & ... Fava, M. (2006). Evaluation of Outcomes with Citalopram for Depression Using Measurement-Based Care in STARD: Implications for Clinical Practice. *American Journal of Psychiatry, 163*(1), 28-40.

Wang, W. & Liang, B. (2012). Case report of mental disorder induced by niacin deficiency. *Shanghai Archives of Psychiatry, 24*(6), 352-254.

# Two

## From Prescription Pad to Health Food Store

As a practitioner of integrative medicine, I treat individuals with a unique array of emotional, behavioral, and physical symptoms. Integrative medicine focuses on the spiritual wellness and physical health of individuals by taking into account of all aspects of their lives. One of the core concepts of Integrative Psychiatry is the understanding of how to increase the body's nutrient reserves to promote long-term health. Lithium is one of the essential nutrients required to achieve optimal health.

Lithium is a naturally occurring element, Number 3 on the Periodic Table. It has been labeled a "Cinderella drug" by Cornell psychiatrist Anna Fels MD because, despite its value, it is neglected and ignored (Fels, 2014). Lithium has not received the attention it deserves. This is partly because it is linked with the stigma of severe mental disorders. The more likely reason is that it is an orphaned treatment because pharmaceutical companies have nothing to gain by marketing or researching an inexpensive element that is available everywhere. It lacks the excitement of novelty and the fanfare of an extravagant launch by a pharmaceutical company.

Nevertheless, I consider lithium the most effective nutritional supplement for neurological and psychiatric disorders. My respect and enthusiasm for lithium treatment may seem surprising considering some of the drug's diverse applications throughout history, its association with severe mental health disorders, and its reputation for side effects. At pharmaceutical doses, lithium is an effective treatment for bipolar disorder, recurrent depression, and suicidal tendencies (Lewitzka et al., 2015). But today many psychiatrists hesitate to prescribe it because of potential side effects at high doses. Their concerns are not unwarranted. Lithium prescribed at pharmaceutical doses can have disabling, irreversible side effects.

I have found that side effects are non-existent, however, when lithium is used as a nutritional supplement. Nutritional lithium is a safe integrative strategy for the treatment of psychiatric and neurological disorders. In fact, it has the potential to dramatically change clinical practice. So instead of pulling out my prescription pad, in most cases I now recommend that patients take lithium as a nutritional supplement. Not only does low dose lithium not have any side effects; it yields tremendous benefits related to many aspects of mood, behavior, and emotional health.

In this book, we will briefly chronicle the history of lithium treatment and present research results on treating and preventing a wide range of neuropsychiatric disorders, including Alzheimer's disease. As my practice has evolved over the past 25 years, I now recommend low dose lithium not only to stabilize mood and help with addictions and impulse control, but also to delay cognitive decline. The book will introduce research that shows how lithium promotes the health, growth, and resilience of neurons. New research now shows that lithium can improve mental health at the genetic level by actually changing the expression of genes. Lithium is an essential part of an integrative, personalized approach to mental health.

## Pharmaceutical vs. Low Dose Lithium

When patients display signs of mania or have suicidal thoughts, pharmaceutical lithium is clearly indicated. I have witnessed dramatic responses to lithium in patients who have suffered from incapacitating mood swings. Some patients were so whipsawed by alternating depression and mania that they could not work or sustain meaningful relationships. In these cases, lithium at pharmaceutical doses—in the range of 600 to 1800 mg—dramatically diminished symptoms.

Yet when prescribed in doses that prove to be too high for an individual patient for an extended period of time, this potentially lifesaving drug can become toxic. Even as it restores patients' emotional lives, it can erode organ systems. Lithium can cause irreversible kidney damage, thyroid disease, tremors, muscle weakness, poor coordination, tinnitus (ringing in the ears), and blurred vision. In a 2014 article in *The New York Times* entitled "I Don't Believe in God, but I Believe in Lithium," writer Jamie Lowe delivers forceful testimony about her own medical dilemma. Lithium, the drug that successfully treated her mania and allowed her to live a normal life, also caused severe kidney damage and placed her at risk of needing a kidney transplant. She stopped lithium, but lived in fear that her manic symptoms would return and sabotage everything she had worked so hard for (Lowe, 2015).

The kidney damage Jamie Lowe suffered is common. Because side effects can be serious, blood levels must be checked regularly in patients taking lithium at pharmaceutical doses. I have found that focusing on patients' blood lithium levels sometimes distracts attention from the disease picture itself. When all emphasis is on monitoring lithium blood levels to attain a "therapeutic range," attention seems to shift from the well-being of the patient to the values in the lab. The question is no longer whether the patient is getting better but whether a certain percentage of lithium is present in his or her blood.

It was not a huge leap for me in 1990 to start exploring the lowest dose of lithium possible that would alleviate my patients' symptoms. Rather than basing my judgment on a number from a lab test, I listened to patients' descriptions of their symptoms. I began to see that patients on a lower dose of lithium—lower than the therapeutic range—still experienced significant clinical benefits.

When I was a student, I came across the work of Jonathan Wright, MD, a Harvard-trained physician who specializes in integrative medicine and nutritional therapies. Jonathan Wright has written about treatment with low dose lithium for almost 30 years. In 1990, after reading about his clinical experience, I prescribed 5 mg of lithium daily for a patient who had struggled with longstanding depression. She got better. Then I began to see bipolar patients who had developed uncomfortable side effects from high doses of lithium and explored whether they could remain free of bipolar symptoms on a lower dose. One of these patients, a 20-year-old woman named Audrey with a history of depression and mood swings and a diagnosis of Bipolar Disease, came to see me because she was experiencing intolerable side effects from the high dose of lithium. When I gradually lowered her dose to 10 mg lithium orotate, she maintained a stable mood and experienced no side effects.

Another case was particularly striking. Paul was a 50-year-old man with severe bipolar disorder. On pharmaceutical doses of lithium he had experienced relief from severe mood swings. But on the high dose, he developed chronic kidney disease secondary to lithium toxicity. After the doctor stopped the lithium, he failed to improve on multiple other medications. He became depressed and unemployed for 3 years. I recommended low dose lithium of 10 mg of lithium orotate per day. Over time, Paul began to feel better, and he returned to work and resumed his regular life activities.

When his kidney specialist heard that Paul was taking lithium again, however, he urged him to stop the nutritional lithium. The symptoms of bipolar disease crept back into his life. Paul began to cycle between moods; his career and personal friendships suffered. Then, without telling either me or his nephrologist, Paul began to titrate lithium orotate himself. Paul found that he could remain free of bipolar symptoms if he took 20 milligrams of lithium orotate a week. This is a very low dose that causes absolutely no harm to organ systems. He has remained free of mood swings while protecting his kidneys from further damage for ten years since starting lithium orotate.

## The Potential of Nutritional Lithium

Even though lithium is among one of the oldest medications in psychiatry, large-scale scientific studies of low dose lithium are limited. Why? Because there is no profit in it. Pharmaceutical companies do not eagerly sponsor studies of inexpensive generic medications. A prescription for lithium costs pennies, and of course, pharmaceutical companies reap no benefit from a nutritional supplement purchased at a health food store.

# Nutritional Lithium: A Cinderella Story

Although they have not been publicized, studies of low dose lithium are not new. Forty years ago, William Walsh, PhD conducted a controlled study comparing lithium concentration in the scalp hair of convicted murderers to lithium concentration in the scalp hair of law-abiding individuals. He found that the convicted killers had only one-third the lithium content in their scalp hair as those who had not broken the law. Eagerly, he took his results to criminology professional societies and to the American Psychiatric Association. But no one paid attention.

Now small observational and interventional studies have positively associated modest concentrations of lithium with mental, emotional, and behavioral benefits. Small randomized, double-blind, placebo-controlled trials have indicated positive emotional and behavioral changes with short-term low dose supplementation with lithium. In one study, 24 participants with histories of aggression and impulsivity took a 4-week course of 40 mcg of lithium daily. At the end of the month, their scores on measures of happiness, friendliness, energy, and mood had improved (Schrauzer & deVroey, 1990). In another study, participants receiving low dose lithium for 12 months experienced statistically significant increases in both memory and attention (Leyhe et al., 2009).

Studies of lithium in the water supply provide enlightening evidence of the benefits of low dose lithium. Low lithium content in the water supply is correlated with higher rates of mental and emotional disorders. In 1970, one research study analyzed levels of organically derived lithium in the water of 27 Texas counties and compared them to the incidence of admissions and readmissions for psychoses, neuroses, and personality disorders at local and state mental hospitals (Schrauzer & Shrestha, 1990). The authors noted a clear trend: the higher the lithium content in the water supply, the lower the rate of psychiatric illness in that county. This association remained significant even after possible confounding variables were accounted for.

Uncertain whether these striking findings were unique to the geographical region, researchers sought to replicate the study in other areas. Lithium water studies have been conducted in Austria, England, Greece, and Japan (Giotakos et al., 2013; Kabacs et al., 2011; Kapusta et al., 2011; Ohgami et al., 2009). Data collection from all of these studies has confirmed a strong inverse correlation between aggressive crime and suicide, and supplemental levels of lithium in the water supply.

The potential of far-reaching use of low dose lithium presents exciting possibilities. In 2014, Anna Fels, MD proposes in her *New York Times* editorial:

> "What if micro-dose lithium were again part of our standard nutritional fare? What if it were added back to soft drinks or popular vitamin brands or even put in the water supply? The research to date strongly suggests that suicide levels could be reduced, and even perhaps other violent acts. And maybe the dementia rate would decline. We don't know because the research hasn't been done" (Fels, 2014).

While decades of research tell us that higher lithium concentration in drinking water is correlated with improved psychological well-being and overall decreased mortality rates, researchers recently found that lithium may also promote longevity in humans (Zarse et al., 2011). They discovered that low dose lithium exposure extended the life span of the model organism, the roundworm *Caenorhabditis elegans*.

As the medical community waits for the results of more research studies, we want not only to help patients who suffer from poorly treated psychiatric and neurological disorders—but also to share our experience in using low dose lithium. Even without an expensive rollout from a pharmaceutical company, health care professionals and patients will see benefits from the use of nutritional lithium. As the research on lithium expands, the message will reach not only patients whose conditions require lithium through a prescription pad, but also those who seek the benefits of this mineral at a health food store. The compelling benefits of low dose lithium therapy provide hope that in the future, you will not have to choose between mental and physical health. With low dose lithium, you can have both.

Lithium is truly a Cinderella treatment: an old, unnoticed treatment with sparkling promise for alleviating human suffering.

## CHAPTER 2 | References

Fels, A. (2014, September 13). Should we all take a bit of lithium? *The New York Times*, pp. 6.

Giotakos, O., Nisianakis, P., Tsouvelas, G., & Giakalou, V.V. (2013). Lithium in the public water supply and suicide mortality in Greece. *Biological Trace Elements Research, 156*(1-3), 376-9.

Kabacs, N., Memon, A., Obinwa, T., Stochl, J., & Perez, J. (2011). Lithium in drinking water and suicide rates across the East of England. *British Journal of Psychiatry, 198*(5), 406-7.

Kapusta, N. D., Mossaheb, N., Etzersdorfer, E., Hlavin, G., Thau, K., Willeit, M., & ... Leithner-Dziubas, K. (2011). Lithium in drinking water and suicide mortality. *British Journal of Psychiatry, 198*(5), 346-350.

Lewitzka, U., Severus, E., Bauer, R., Ritter, P., Müller-Oerlinghausen, B., & Bauer, M. (2015). The suicide prevention effect of lithium: more than 20 years of evidence-a narrative review. *International Journal of Bipolar Disorders, 3*(1), 32.

Leyhe, T., Eschweiler, G. W., Stransky, E., Gasser, T., Annas, P., Basun, H., & Laske, C. (2009). Increase of BDNF serum concentration in lithium treated patients with early Alzheimer's disease. *Journal oOf Alzheimer's Disease, 16*(3), 649-656.

Lowe, J. (2015, June 28). 'I Don't Believe in God, but I Believe in Lithium'. *The New York Times Magazine*, pp. 54.

Ohgami, H., Terao, T., Shiotsuki, I., Ishii, N., & Iwata, N. (2009). Lithium levels in drinking water and risk of suicide. *British Journal of Psychiatry, 194*(5), 464-5.

Raloff, J. (1983). Locks: A Key to Violence? *Science News, 124*(8), 122-125.

Schrauzer, G. N., & deVroey, E. (1994). Effects of nutritional lithium supplementation on mood. A placebo-controlled study with former drug users. *Biological Trace Element Research, 40*(1), 89-101.

Schrauzer, G.N. & Shrestha, K.P. (1990). Lithium in drinking water and the incidences of crimes, suicides, and arrests related to drug addictions. *Biological Trace Elements Research, 25*(2), 105-13.

Zarse, K., Terao, T., Tian, J., Iwata, N., Ishii, N., & Ristow, M. (2011). Low-dose lithium uptake promotes longevity in humans and metazoans. *European Journal of Nutrition, 50*(5), 387-389.

# Three

## THE HISTORY OF LITHIUM: HOW A MINERAL BECOMES A MEDICINE

Even the soft drink entrepreneur Charles Leiper Grigg understood there was something special about lithium. In 1929, he unveiled a drink called Bib-Label Lithiated Lemon-Lime Soda with the slogan "It takes the ouch out of the grouch." Hailed for improving mood and curing hangovers, this product was eventually rechristened 7-Up. The "7" supposedly represents the rounded-up atomic weight of the element lithium (6.9), and the "Up'" suggests its power to lift spirits. Lithium remained an ingredient of 7-Up until 1950 (El-Mallakh & Roberts, 2007).

Centuries before the advent of this celebrated soft drink, lithium was associated with calming moods. Soranus, a physician from ancient Ephesus, observed the benefits of alkaline springs for soothing the wild spirits of some of his patients. Lithium, it turned out, was abundant in these springs (Georgotas & Gershon, 1981).

Natural springs containing lithium were popular in both the Eastern and the Western hemispheres through the nineteenth century. Archaeology unearthed evidence that Lithia Springs, Georgia was a sacred Cherokee Indian site. That the site remained respected is clear from records showing that several American Presidents, including Cleveland, Taft, McKinley, and Theodore

# The History of Lithium: How A Mineral Becomes A Medicine

Roosevelt, visited Lithia Springs in search of a health cure. In 1890, the Lithia Springs Sanitarium was established to treat compulsive behaviors including alcoholism and opioid dependence (Georgotas & Gershon, 1981).

The simple element lithium, which is plentiful in alkaline springs, gets its name from the Greek word for stone, *lithos*. Lithium is unevenly distributed on the earth. In addition to its presence in natural springs, lithium is found in granite and other rocks as well as in sea water. When rocks break down, lithium leaches into the soil, where it is readily absorbed by plants and enters the food chain. The most common source of lithium in the modern diet is tap water (Schrauzer, 2002). Medical use of lithium was first publicized by London doctor Alfred Baring Garrod in treating patients with gout. After discovering uric acid in the blood of his gout patients, he wrote about pioneering the use of lithium in his 1859 treatise, *The Nature and Treatment of Gout and Rheumatic Gout* (Strobusch, 1980).

For several decades lithium tablets and other products containing lithium were recommended for treating kidney and bladder problems as well as gallstones. The Sears, Roebuck & Company Catalogue of 1908 advertised Schieffelin's Effervescent Lithia Tablets for a variety of afflictions. By 1907, The *Merck Index* listed 43 different medicinal preparations containing lithium. Excitement about these lithium products reflected the predominant view that uric acid caused a plethora of diseases, including headache, epilepsy, depression, melancholia, suicide, high blood pressure, angina, asthma, Raynaud's disease, gout and rheumatism. As the popularity of the uric acid explanation for disease declined, interest in lithium products waned (Strobusch, 1980).

It was in Denmark where lithium was first used to treat mood disorders. Two psychiatrist brothers, Fredrik and Carl Lange, reported in the first Danish textbook of clinical psychiatry that they had successfully used lithium in patients with depression. The patients' symptoms, often suicidal thoughts or poor impulse control, resolved while they were taking lithium but often returned after they were discharged. The Langes therefore tried to continue lithium therapy with those patients after they left the hospital (Bech, 2007). With the death of Frederik Lange in 1907, the use of lithium in treating mood disorders was forgotten. During the first half of the twentieth century, there are virtually no references to lithium in the psychiatric literature (Bech, 2007).

# Nutritional Lithium: A Cinderella Story

The twentieth century revival of lithium as a psychiatric remedy began in 1949 in Melbourne, Australia, with John Cade, who knew of Garrod's success in lithium treatment a century before. As a Japanese prisoner of war a few years earlier, he had noticed that the disruptive and impulsive behaviors of some of his fellow prisoners subsided after they urinated. He speculated that an excess of uric acid might underlie his patients' mania, and he began treating them with lithium. Some responded strikingly well, even after years of illness and unsuccessful treatment with other medications (Cade, 1949). Although published in an obscure journal, Cade's article described a well-designed and executed research study and focused on the rational presentation of results rather than rhapsodizing about the virtues of a particular treatment. Because of his well-structured study and the dramatic treatment results, some historians of medicine consider that John Cade ushered in modern psychopharmacology.

Unfortunately, the timing of Cade's treatment successes was unfortunate. The very same year, 1949, adverse reaction reports surfaced in the media about patients who were taking lithium in a different form for a completely different purpose. As physicians in the U.S. encouraged their patients with heart disease and hypertension to avoid sodium chloride, lithium chloride was marketed as an alternative. In the early 1950s, physicians released reports of patients who developed lithium poisoning after they had consumed large amounts of lithium chloride. Several deaths were reported, leading the FDA to ban the use of lithium salt substitutes. "Stop using this dangerous poisoning at once!" exhorted the FDA. Unsurprisingly, lithium again fell out of favor with the medical community (Strobusch, 1980).

Despite the lithium chloride debacle, Cade's study prompted a few isolated studies of lithium in Australia and in France. The next breakthrough happened again in Denmark. Psychiatrist Mogens Schou, who read Cade's article, tried an entirely new research design: a randomized controlled trial. This experiment would study the effectiveness of lithium for treating mania by randomizing manic patients—literally by tossing a coin—to receive either lithium or placebo. Schou's experiment revealed that 70% of patients with mania responded to lithium. Schou introduced the term "mood normalizer" to convey lithium's ability to stabilize abnormal mood swings while not affecting normal emotions in the ways that amphetamines and barbiturates do.

# The History of Lithium: How A Mineral Becomes A Medicine

Charting the natural history of bipolar disorder, with its predictable recurrences and progressive character, he demonstrated lithium's beneficial effects not only as a maintenance drug but also as preventive medication (Shorter, 2009).

The U.S. was slow to embrace and fund the study of lithium. Several case reports of side effects from lithium treatment, including slurred speech and hypertension, constitute the early literature (Solomon & Vickers, 1975). But gradually a "lithium underground" formed of physicians prescribing lithium in the absence of official FDA approval. Finally, in 1970, the U.S. was the 50th country to approve lithium for treatment of acute mania. In 1974, lithium was also approved to prevent recurrent mania (Shorter, 2009).

There followed an upsurge in prescriptions for lithium to treat patients for acute mania and to prevent relapse of both manic and depressive cycles in bipolar disorder. Lithium was established as the first-line treatment for bipolar disorder. Despite the impressive effectiveness of lithium in clinical trials, the fortunes of lithium again shifted into decline in the mid 1990's. When newer medications like valproate came on the market, lithium lost its ascendancy as the first-line treatment for bipolar disorder (Shorter, 2009).

Lithium has undergone a shifting and dramatic history in medicine, sometimes celebrated as a panacea, sometimes reviled as toxic, sometimes totally forgotten before reappearing in scientific experiments in another country in another context. Still, after the intervening centuries and billion dollar pharmaceutical breakthroughs, no drug has superseded lithium for stabilizing mood and preventing suicide in patients with bipolar disorder. It seems paradoxical that after decades that have witnessed release of new and expensive pharmaceutical products, the best results for patients with mood disorders are achieved through psychiatry's oldest medication that is simply a mineral essential for brain health.

## Lithium in Manufacturing and Technology

No history of lithium's uses would be complete without acknowledging the element's importance to the world of manufacturing and technology. Only about 5% of the world's lithium supply is actually used for health-related purposes. The remaining 95% is used in industry.

# Nutritional Lithium: A Cinderella Story

Lithium is extracted from the earth by two different methods: mining lithium ores and mining lithium brines in salt lakes. Beginning in the late 1990's, brines became the main source because processing hard rock ore is more expensive. Brine deposits, which represent about 66% of the global lithium supply, are found mainly in the salt flats of Chile, Argentina, China, and Tibet. There is only one brine operation in the United States (U.S. Geological Survey, 2015).

Recent high demand for lithium in industry has led to increased mining and production. Both Argentina and Chile increased their production of lithium about 15% in 2014, and the brine operation in the U.S. recently doubled its former capacity (U.S. Geological Survey, 2015). Lithium's properties ensure many uses in technology. The lightest of all solid elements, lithium is strong yet highly reactive, malleable, and a good conductor of heat and electricity. For many years, lithium compounds have been used in the production of ceramics, glass, and aluminum products. Because of lithium, Corning and Pyrex cookware, for instance, can be moved from refrigerator to oven without shattering. Lithium helps decrease thermal expansion and increase shock resistance (O'Bannon, 1984).

Lithium in varied forms has a broad range of industrial applications. As a metal, lithium is commonly used for aircraft parts because of its lightness. Lithium aluminum and lithium magnesium alloys are strong even at high temperatures and have considerable tensile strength. Lithium is in greatest demand for use in batteries. Its advantages include low weight, high energy density, and high electric output per weight. Unlike nickel batteries, lithium batteries do not lose energy if they are charged before being fully depleted.

Lithium batteries have become popular in aerospace because they are virtually maintenance-free. The Mars Curiosity Rover uses lithium nickel oxide cells that are only partially charged and discharged. Under this system, the life span is four years (Buchmann, 2011). Lithium sulfur dioxide batteries were essential to the Mars Exploration Rovers Spirit and Opportunity. The batteries successfully supported the entry, descent, and landing and preserved enough energy for post-landing operations (Ratnakumar, 2004).

Lithium has also drawn the attention of automotive manufacturers in their quest to develop environmentally friendly vehicles. Toyota, Honda, Nissan,

# The History of Lithium: How A Mineral Becomes A Medicine

Ford, and other automotive companies have produced successful prototype cars using lithium batteries. As battery production increases, costs decrease (Western Lithium Corporation, n.d.). By 2017, Tesla is planning to release its Model 3 car, which is expected to cost only $30,000 and to drive more than a 200-mile range between charges. General Motors has promised to release a similar car in 2017. Analysts speculate that by 2020, several million electric battery-based cars will be on the road (Hunt, 2015). The lithium batteries that will power them have the potential to revolutionize transportation while not harming the environment.

Plans are now underway for a new highway to connect the only remaining American lithium mine, in Silver Peak, Nevada, to a large Tesla factory. By 2020, this factory alone is expected projected to produce more lithium batteries annually than were produced worldwide in 2013. Lithium has a host of other technical uses, both simple and complex. When fireworks colored red light up the night sky, lithium is responsible (Johanson, 2007). The Apollo 13 astronauts relied on canisters containing powdered lithium hydroxide to remove carbon dioxide from their spacecraft atmosphere (NASA, 2009).

The history of lithium has followed an amazing trajectory: from the calming springs of ancient Ephesus to the sophisticated technology of the space age. Lithium is revolutionizing aspects of technology, from batteries to automobiles, airplanes to space vehicles. Demand for lithium is on the rise because of its versatility, light weight, conductivity, high energy density, and malleability. Some economists predict that lithium supply will soon drive the economy. This shape-shifting element clearly has a future beyond its applications in health and disease.

## CHAPTER 3 | References

Bech, P. (2007). The full story of lithium. *Nordic Journal of Psychiatry, 61*(46), 35-39.

Buchmann, I. (2011). *Batteries in the Industrial Market.* Cadex Electronics Inc. Retrieved from www.batteryuniversity.com/learn/article/batteries_for_medical_consumer_hobbyist

Cade, J. J. (1949). Lithium salts in the treatment of psychotic excitement. *Medical Journal of Australia, 2*(10), 349-352.

El-Mallakh, R. S., & Roberts, R. J. (2007). Lithiated lemon-lime sodas. *American Journal of Psychiatry, 164*(11), 1662.

Georgotas, A., Gershon, S. 1981. Historical perspectives and current highlights on lithium treatment in manic-depressive illness. *Journal of Clinical Psychopharmacology, 1*(1), 27-31.

Hunt, Tam. (2015). *The Geopolitics of Lithium Production.* Greentech Media. Retrieved from www.greentechmedia.com/articles/read/the-geopolitics-of-lithium-production

Johanson, P. (2007). *Lithium.* New York, NY: Rosen Publishing Group, Inc.

NASA. (2009). *Apollo 13.* Retrieved from www.nasa.gov/mission_pages/apollo/missions/apollo13.html

O'Bannon, Loran S. (1984). *Dictionary of Ceramic Science and Engineering.* New York, NY: Plenum Press. pp. 156.

Ratnakumar, B. V. (2004). *Lithium-sulfur dioxide batteries on Mars rovers.* Pasadena, CA: Jet Propulsion Laboratory, National Aeronautics and Space Administration.

Schrauzer, G. N. (2002). Lithium: occurrence, dietary intakes, nutritional essentiality. *Journal of the American College of Nutrition, 21*(1), 14-21.

Shorter, E. (2009). The history of lithium therapy. *Bipolar Disorders, 11*(Suppl. 2), 4-9.

Solomon, K., & Vickers, R. (1975). Dysarthria resulting from lithium carbonate. A case report. *JAMA, 231*(3), 280.

# The History of Lithium: How A Mineral Becomes A Medicine

Strobusch, A. D., & Jefferson, J. W. (1980). The Checkered History of Lithium in Medicine. *Pharmacy in History*, 22(2), 72-76.

Jaskula, B. (2015). *Mineral Commodity Summaries.* U.S. Geological Survey. Retrieved from http://minerals.usgs.gov/minerals/pubs/commodity/lithium/mcs-2015-lithi.pdf

# Four

## Nutritional Lithium as a Dietary Supplement

While the use of lithium in the treatment of manic depressive illness known as bipolar disorder remains a gold standard treatment today, many do not think about lithium as an essential mineral critical for human health. There are significant inconsistencies in international regulations. Countries including Canada, the United Kingdom, Taiwan, and the Philippines prohibit the sale of nutritional lithium because it is only recognized as a pharmaceutical. The use of lithium is also highly controlled in Japan. In Austria, nutritional supplements are restricted from containing any lithium salts. The only way to obtain nutritional lithium would be to ingest it through diet or a lithium-rich source, such as a special plant extract. The United States and Hong Kong allow the sale of lithium as a nutritional supplement.

It is quite clear that one of the major challenges preventing widespread use of nutritional lithium is the overall perception of it—that it is a medication with side effects. However, lithium is an essential mineral for health and emotional well-being. Scientists now suggest a provisional Recommended Daily Allowance of lithium 1 mg per day per 70 kg (154 lbs.) for adults (Schrauzer, 2002). Because the Recommended Daily Allowance only describes the minimum requirement to meet the needs of healthy individuals, 1 mg per day may not be sufficient for those who require additional support. The following chapters will discuss how an individual's genetic and epigenetic profile interacting with environmental stressors may reflect a need for higher doses of lithium to achieve optimal brain function.

## Pharmaceutical Lithium

In the United States, lithium carbonate and lithium citrate are approved for the treatment of bipolar disorder. All but the extended-release tablets are often taken three times a day to maintain a constant serum concentration of lithium. All forms are taken orally with food, and lithium is absorbed by the body through the same mechanism as other minerals.

Lithium travels from the stomach into the small intestines, where it is rapidly absorbed into the bloodstream. As the blood travels to the brain, it is actively transported across the blood-brain barrier. Although the exact mechanism is unclear, researchers hypothesize that lithium ions concentrate outside of the cell membrane, causing depolarization of the neuron, where gated ion channels on the cell membrane open to allow sodium to rush into the cell. Because of lithium's similarity in molecular structure and charge to sodium, lithium can easily displace sodium ions and cross the blood-brain barrier instead. Lithium is most effective if it is maintained at a constant level in the body, and a consistent amount of salt is present in the diet. Imbalances in fluid and salt levels affect serum concentrations of lithium, and dehydration can result in toxicity.

The lowest prescription strength is available as 150 mg tablets. The liquid preparation of lithium carbonate is available at 300 mg per 5 milliliters (mL) or 1 tablespoon. Until recently, most psychiatrists were trained to start lithium at 300 mg twice daily and increase to a therapeutic blood level ignoring total dosage. Psychiatrists prescribe lithium for a total prescription dose range between 600 to 1800 mg per day. Routine blood tests are required to monitor lithium levels in the blood to prevent lithium toxicity. Lithium medications are often sold under the brand names Eskalith, Lithonate, Lithobid, and Lithium Carbonate ER.

Most patients who are on maintenance therapy are stabilized with at least 900 mg daily. However, patients who are experiencing acute mania are maintained with up to 1800 mg per day. These doses will normally produce the desired serum lithium level of 1.0 to 1.5 mEq/L. Lithium carbonate can become toxic due to the poor bioavailability of the carrier salt, which causes lithium to accumulate in the blood. Lithium carbonate increases extracellular lithium levels, requiring elevated levels in order for it to enter cells to be absorbed.

Unfortunately, the therapeutic index of prescription lithium is narrow, with an acceptable range of 0.6 to 1.5 mEq/L. The optimal concentration of lithium for maintenance treatment of bipolar disorder is generally considered to fall between 0.6 to 1.2 mEq/L, and toxicity can occur at levels greater than 1.5 mEq/L (Finley et al., 1995). At serum concentrations above 1.5 mEq/L, adverse side effects including gastrointestinal complaints, tremors, confusion, and somnolence have been reported. At levels greater than 2.5 mEq/L, seizure and death can occur (McKnight et al., 2012). For many patients, however, nutritional lithium is a safe and simple alternative.

## Nutritional Lithium

Low doses of lithium, at a fraction of the pharmacological dose, can be purchased without a prescription in some health food stores across the U.S. While the regulations regarding sale of nutritional lithium vary widely across the globe, lithium supplements are recognized as a dietary food by the U.S. Food and Drug Administration. Lithium supplements are generally prepared and dispensed as capsules, tablets, or liquid solutions. Lithium supplements are also available in different forms, as lithium must be compounded with a mineral carrier in order for the body to safely absorb it. Popular mineral transporters include citrate, orotate, and aspartate.

Nutritional lithium is intended to supplement the diet and does not require routine blood tests to establish a therapeutic level. With nutritional lithium, there is no "therapeutic window", and many patients can benefit from low doses without concerns about adverse side effects or toxicity.

Lithium aspartate and lithium orotate are available as capsules, and lithium citrate and lithium chloride are available as liquid solutions for purchase without a doctor's prescription. I recommend lithium orotate or lithium citrate for nutritional supplementation. Aspartate belongs in a class of chemicals known as *excitotoxins*, which causes neurons to transmit impulses at such a rapid rate that the receptors quickly become exhausted. The overstimulation can cause unwanted problems such as headaches and possible inflammation in sensitive individuals.

Lithium orotate contains a salt derived from orotic acid that is frequently used as a binder for many mineral supplements. The orotate ion allows lithium to pass through the stomach while remaining bound to the orotate carrier. Blood levels peak between a half hour and two hours after ingestion. Once in the bloodstream, lithium travels to the brain. Based on research on the absorption of calcium and magnesium orotate, lithium orotate is thought to use passive transport to cross the blood-brain barrier. Because the lithium remains attached to the orotate carrier, it directly enters neural cells before being released, leaving little left in the bloodstream to cause unwanted side effects.

Smith and Schou conducted an experiment to compare the therapeutic profile between lithium orotate and lithium carbonate. They injected orotate and carbonate into different groups of mice and measured the lithium concentrations in the blood, kidney, and heart. They found that a smaller amount of lithium orotate is required to achieve the same effect as lithium carbonate, and advised caution when considering high doses of lithium orotate (Smith & Schou, 1979). In regards to the safety and side effect profile of lithium orotate, the authors also concluded that despite lithium orotate's potency, impaired kidney function did not result in the animal study.

Lithium carbonate contains 18.8 mg of elemental lithium per 100 mg. Most lithium orotate compounds contain 3.83 mg of elemental lithium per 100 mg. Lithium orotate does not contain enough elemental lithium per recommended dosage to cause lithium serum concentrations to advance beyond therapeutic levels. The amount of lithium that enters the bloodstream does not reach toxic levels when bound to orotate since all of the lithium enters the cells and does not remain in the extracellular fluid (Nieper, 1973).

Lithium is quickly excreted from the body so multiple doses are needed each day to maintain a therapeutic level. About 95% of lithium is excreted via the kidneys and the other 5% is excreted via saliva, sweat, and feces. Lithium is excreted unchanged in the urine. There are two phases of renal excretion:

rapid clearance of up to two-thirds within 6-12 hours, then a slower elimination over the next twelve hours. The overall half-life is between 12 and 24 hours.

In the 1970's, Dr. Nieper treated 64 patients who suffered from migraine headaches, depression, alcoholism, and epilepsy with lithium orotate. He observed them for up to two and a half years and found that lithium orotate is effective at low doses, causes no negative side effects, and is more effective than lithium citrate and lithium carbonate (Nieper, 1973). Dr. Nieper's key contribution was to show that the orotate and aspartate forms of lithium enabled significantly more lithium to become intracellular, whereas lithium carbonate delivered mostly extracellular lithium.

Research demonstrates that lower doses of lithium orotate are capable of achieving therapeutic brain lithium concentrations while avoiding toxicity and ensuring stable blood concentrations when compared to lithium carbonate (Kling et al., 1978). The dose response and time course for lithium concentrations in the blood and brain were monitored in a group of mice. At each dose, the blood and brain lithium concentrations were greater after orotate than carbonate. After 24 hours, brain lithium concentrations were about three times greater with orotate than carbonate. A subsequent study exploring the effects of lithium orotate in the treatment of alcoholism also found lithium orotate effective in much lower doses than carbonate and citrate, minimizing the possibility of impaired renal impairment (Sartori, 1986).

## Determining Supplementation of Lithium

In 1985, the US Environmental Protection Agency estimated that Americans consume between 0.6 to 3.1 milligrams of lithium per day through water, vegetables, and grains (Schrauzer, 2002). Lithium deficiency is an established but poorly described phenomenon that appears to impact the central nervous system function.

Although there are several factors that determine whether an individual may benefit from low dose lithium, I emphasize focusing primarily on clinical history, family history, and whether a lithium deficiency is detected through a Hair Tissue Mineral Analysis (HTMA). These factors enable me to determine which patients will likely benefit from nutritional lithium supplementation.

### CLINICAL HISTORY

Lithium is helpful in treating a wide range of psychiatric and neurological symptoms. It has been shown to have incredible value as a nutritional supplement for mood disorders. I often see individuals who struggle with uncontrollable mood swings and experience periods of depression benefit from low dose lithium ranging between 5 to 30 milligrams per day.

From a detailed clinical history, I have found that the presence of one symptom—irritability—almost guarantees that nutritional lithium will help. If a patient reports feeling irritable, either as a symptom by itself or as part of a mood disorder diagnosis, I consider this a clear indication for treatment with nutritional lithium.

Other symptoms or related diagnoses that suggest that an individual may be a good candidate for low dose lithium include:

*Anger/Aggression.* I always consider low dose lithium when treating patients who struggle with any aspect of anger and rage. This can manifest as snapping with annoyance at family members, to committing acts of emotional abuse toward children and spouses, to domestic violence.

*Mood Disorders.* Lithium has great value as a nutritional supplement for stabilizing moods. The intensity of cycles of sadness and depression alternating with bouts of aggression and rage can usually be diminished by a nutritional dose of lithium. Patients who have experienced poor responses to antidepressants in the past tend to benefit from lithium. Nutritional lithium can be added to any antidepressant medication or supplement protocol.

*Attention-Deficit Hyperactivity Disorder (ADHD).* I also find low dose lithium helps with treatment of certain forms of ADHD in patients ranging from early childhood to late adulthood. It provides most help to patients who experience periods of irritability and rage in addition to more typical symptoms of inattention and hyperactivity.

*Addictions and Substance Abuse.* Low dose lithium helps patients who need nutritional and metabolic support to stop abusing alcohol or other drugs. I advise patients to take a nutritional dose of lithium in addition to other nutritional and/or medical interventions. Usually, patients find that lithium supports their moods and helps impulse control to maintain sobriety and avoid relapse.

*Anxiety.* There is a subset of individuals with anxiety and obsessive compulsive disorders that experience dramatic improvement in symptoms while taking nutritional lithium. With patients who present with anxiety symptoms and also have a family history of substance abuse and addiction, lithium often provides dramatic relief for longstanding discomfort not responsive to other medications.

*Eating Disorders.* Anorexia Nervosa is a life-threatening illness that is characterized by restricted intake of food with distorted body image and fears of weight gain. Research and years of clinical experience have demonstrated that lithium provides a unique role in establishing mood regulation and decreased anxiety. Lithium supplements have also been helpful in treating bulimia and binge eating disorder. These eating disorders are characterized by poor impulse control, and lithium often provides enhanced ability to control behavior and improve moods.

*Cognitive Decline and Alzheimer's.* Low dose lithium has been shown to have neuroprotective and neurogenerative properties in patients suffering from Alzheimer's disease and other cognitive impairments. Lithium is also capable of modulating many of the hallmark features of Alzheimer's disease, including decreasing plaques and tangles.

*Other Medical Disorders.* Research has demonstrated how lithium can improve symptoms in a vast majority of medical disorders, including Lyme disease, headaches, and hyperthyroidism. Recent research also shows how lithium is effective at minimizing the cognitive side effects caused by chemotherapy.

## *Family History*

Family history is an important aspect and effective parameter for determining whether nutritional lithium may be beneficial for a patient. In my experience, a family history of any major psychiatric illness or suicide is a strong indicator of a patient who will likely benefit from low dose lithium. Almost invariably, when a patient reports a family history involving severe substance abuse or psychiatric illness in a parent, even if the patient herself is free of these serious symptoms, lithium is likely to help improve her mood.

A detailed family history is often the most important part of any assessment, as it can reveal genetic liabilities for mental illness among other valuable information that is not always discussed. A family history needs to include at least two generations of relatives from both sides of the family to properly identify any patterns of psychiatric illness or suicide. Suicide in any genetically-related family member is a strong clinical indicator of whether an individual would benefit from nutritional lithium. The clinician needs to remember that family members who struggle with depression, substance abuse, or suicidal thoughts are often reluctant to disclose information due to the shame and stigma surrounding mental illness.

## *Hair Tissue Mineral Analysis (HTMA)*

One of the most reliable ways to test lithium levels in the body is through a Hair Tissue Mineral Analysis (HTMA). Hair Tissue Mineral Analysis is a simple, inexpensive, and non-invasive procedure that can evaluate long-term patterns of lithium storage in the body. Hair testing can be done from the comfort of home, and does not require any special laboratory equipment or handling instructions.

Using a clean pair of scissors, hair is collected in small portions from five different locations of the scalp, including the nape of the neck, posterior vertex, and posterior temporal regions. Approximately 100 milligrams of hair sample is submitted to a lab through regular postal mail for analysis, which takes approximately 3-4 weeks. The laboratory report assesses levels and ratios of minerals including lithium, zinc, copper, and magnesium, as well as levels of toxic chemicals such as arsenic, lead, and mercury.

A hair analysis is a reliable indicator of lithium deficiency, because hair is one of the many places that the body eliminates minerals and heavy metals. Hair analyses reflect the status of bioavailable lithium for an average period of two to three months prior, rather than the snapshot plasma would demonstrate (Kronemann et al., 1983). The individual mineral levels, ratios, and patterns of minerals deposited in the hair can reveal how well the body is functioning at a cellular level, as minerals are involved in the body's enzymatic reactions (Watts, 1990). Lithium levels are also higher in hair than blood, making it easier to detect and measure (Adams et al., 2006).

Lithium levels in tissue analysis are important because one can have normal levels in the blood serum sample, but fail to detect high levels in the tissue since lithium can be stored in body tissue. Since hair is a soft tissue, hair analysis can reveal higher levels that might not be detected in other biological samples.

Another way that serum lithium levels may be misleading was found in a study conducted by Schrauzer and colleagues in 2002. Researchers found that in humans supplemented with lithium, serum levels increased proportionally to lithium intake. However, when animals were fed lithium-deficient diets, they did not exhibit differences in their plasma concentrations, suggesting that blood is a poor biomarker for detecting physiological concentrations of lithium. Blood tests are unreliable at detecting a physiological deficiency of lithium.

The methodology for preparing and analyzing samples has been published, and recent studies from around the world have used the same CLIA-certified laboratory, supporting internal validity (Druyan et al., 1998; Schofer & Schrauzer, 2011). The hair collection kit provides step-by-step instructions for the collection of the hair (e.g., the one inch closest to the scalp, stainless steel scissors), supporting uniformity in collection techniques between individuals. Researchers have been publishing on lithium levels obtained through hair analysis since 1975, and thus 16 populations from around the world are available for crude comparison, including temporal trends in lithium levels.

The results from a hair tissue mineral analysis, along with a detailed clinical and family history, can offer tremendous insight about the clinical utility of low dose lithium therapy for individuals. I recommend nutritional lithium for any patient who presents with one or more of these factors.

## Nutritional Lithium Dosage

For any healthy individual seeking optimal health, I recommend 2 to 5 milligrams of lithium orotate per day. For individuals over the age of 40, I would increase the supplemental dosage to 5 to 10 milligrams per day to counteract the cognitive decline associated with the aging process. For patients who require symptom reduction, I recommend dose ranges between 5 to 40 mg of lithium orotate.

Effects from low dose lithium supplementation are often seen within 2 to 4 weeks, but there are no established protocols that determine how much of the nutritional supplement one should take. Each individual has his or her own unique biochemical needs, and dosage for nutritional lithium should be titrated slowly to identify the optimal dose. Some people have reported feeling significantly better on only 2 milligrams per day, while some reported feeling too subdued or "flat" on 5 milligrams. Every individual is different, and patients should work with their health care provider to determine their own optimal dose.

## Monitoring Lithium Supplementation

Despite the low risks associated with nutritional doses of lithium, anyone interested in taking lithium supplements should be monitored by a health professional. Before initiating low dose lithium, I also screen for the presence of any thyroid disorders, which are becoming increasingly common among the US population, where an estimated 20 million people are affected.

The anti-thyroid effects of lithium were first studied in detail when patients who were treated with lithium carbonate developed hypothyroidism and goiter, an abnormal enlargement of the thyroid gland. Animal and human studies later revealed that lithium increases intrathyroidal iodine content by inhibiting the coupling of iodotyrosine residues to form thyroxine [T4] and triiodothyronine [T3] (Bagchi et al., 1978). Thyroid hormones can affect energy level, mood, and behavior. Subclinical hypothyroidism (normal T4 with raised TSH) occurs in up to 40 percent of patients with mood disorders. Low thyroid function has also been linked to poorer responses to treatment for mood disorders with lower rates of recovery. It is important to ensure that patients who are taking lithium supplements do not have undiagnosed hypothyroidism.

Although I have rarely detected lithium blood levels with patients taking lithium orotate, I recommend checking serum lithium levels after 3 months of initiating lithium supplementation. Renal, parathyroid, and thyroid function tests can be evaluated yearly. Women who are looking to become pregnant while receiving lithium should be advised about the possible risk of congenital malformation. They should also discuss their intentions to conceive with their physician before initiating lithium therapy.

## Side Effects of Nutritional Lithium Supplementation

For over 25 years, I have prescribed nutritional lithium and have not observed any adverse effects. Rarely, patients prescribed nutritional lithium report feeling "too subdued" or "too relaxed" to the extent they feel uncomfortable. When lithium is discontinued, these symptoms are resolved.

There has been one published case report discussing side effects from nutritional lithium, which include hand tremors, nausea, vomiting, excessive thirst, and frequent urination. This case study was published in 2009 involving an 18-year-old female who presented in the emergency department after consuming 18 tablets of 120 mg of lithium orotate (Pauze & Brooks, 2007). She complained of nausea, emesis, and a mild tremor. After she received intravenous fluids and an anti-emetic, her nausea and tremor were resolved and her serum lithium level was well below the accepted range.

According to Jonathan Wright, MD, one of the most experienced practitioners and leading advocates for low dose lithium, a total daily intake of 30 milligrams of elemental lithium will not have any noticeable effects on serum lithium levels, and up to 40 milligrams appears to be completely safe, with no negative side effects or signs of toxicity. He has found these doses to be effective in his patients with a variety of mental, neurological, and physical conditions.

Although adverse side effects seldom occur with sub-pharmaceutical doses of lithium, I always recommend that anyone taking lithium also take essential fatty acids along with vitamin E to minimize the possibility of side effects. Lithium is known to inhibit the synthesis of prostaglandin E1 by blocking the mobilization of dihomogammalinolenic acid (DGLA), and lithium toxicity may be related to decreased prostaglandin formation. Therefore, patients with a functional essential fatty acid deficiency may be at risk of developing side effects while receiving lithium therapy (Manku et al, 1979).

In one report, supplementation with essential fatty acids in the form of safflower oil (3 to 5 grams per day) reversed symptoms of prescription lithium toxicity such as tremor and ataxia (Lieb, 1980). Essential fatty acids are important adjuncts to treatment of lithium's side effects, so consuming extra quantities of essential fatty acids may eliminate the possibility of side effects.

Another concern with lithium use is the possibility of thyroid dysfunction. Zinc is a key mineral that serves as a cofactor in the production of thyroid releasing hormone (TRH) in the brain. TRH is responsible for sending a signal to the pituitary to synthesize thyroid stimulating hormone (TSH)

(Pekary et al., 1991). Because zinc can be depleted by stress, heavy sweating, and vegetarianism, adequate zinc is needed to prevent thyroid damage. In one study, researchers found that zinc supplementation was able to protect and normalize thyroid function following 4 months of lithium therapy (Li, Li, & Li, 2015). For patients who are on nutritional lithium, I also recommend a minimum of 30-60 mg of zinc daily to prevent possible side effects.

## Dosage for Nutritional Lithium

While the data on the dosage of nutritional lithium is lacking, doses as low as 400 micrograms have been found to improve mental health outcomes in a research study of patients with a history of substance abuse (Shrauzer & de Vroey, 1994). The symptoms of lithium deficiency and toxicity can be visualized as a theoretical U-shaped curve where either state can result in health problems (Mischley, 2012).

In Figure 4.1, the graph highlights the deficiency zone, where individuals who receive less than 1 mg of elemental lithium per day will experience symptoms of deficiency, including aggressive behavior, diminished impulse control, mood lability, and increased suicidal thoughts. As the lithium dose increases toward the pharmacological range of 600 to 2000 mg per day, symptoms associated with bipolar disorder, depression, and possible dystonia can appear (Figure 4.2). At pharmacological doses greater than 2000 mg per day, as shown in Figure 4.3, symptoms of lithium toxicity including gastrointestinal complaints, tremors, confusion, seizure, and possibly death may occur. It appears that many environmental and genetic influences affect the maintenance dose as highlighted in Figure 4.4. At sub-pharmaceutical doses, lithium is found to improve cell growth, enhance electrolyte regulation across neuron membranes, and support neuronal health.

## Nutritional Lithium: A Cinderella Story

**Figure 4.1**
Lithium deficiency

**Figure 4.2**
Pharmacological doses of lithium

**Figure 4.3**
Lithium toxicity

**Figure 4.4**
Maintenance dose to support neuronal health

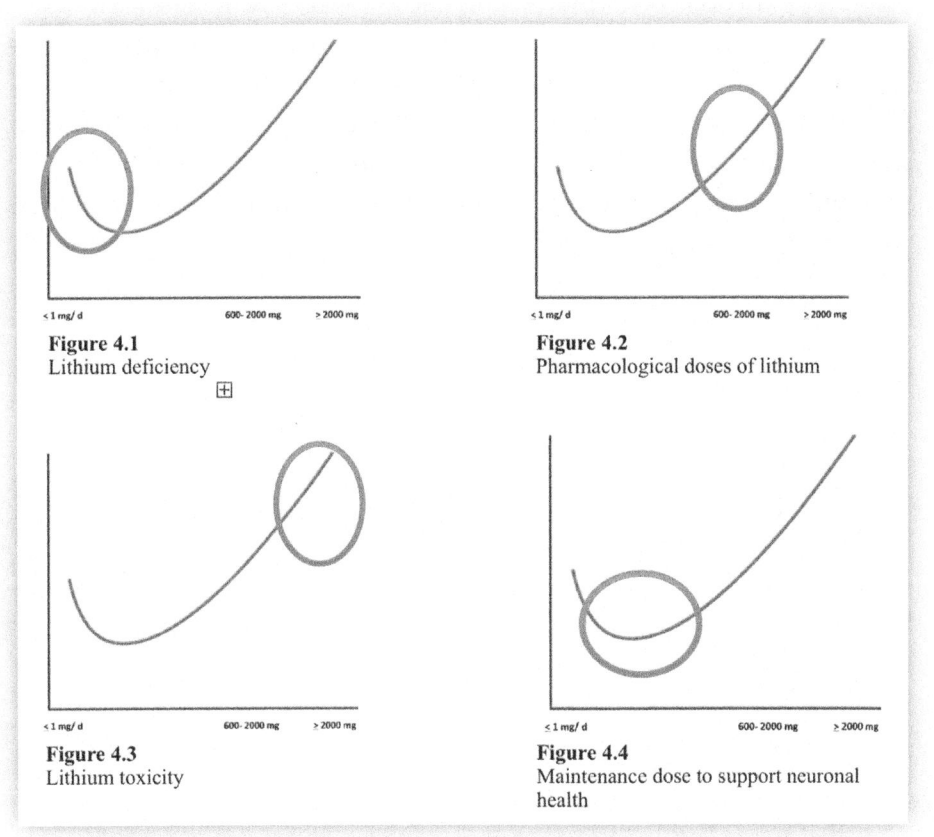

*Figures 4.1 to 4.4.* Adapted from "The Role of Lithium in Central Nervous System Health," by Laurie K. Mischley, Presented at the 43rd Orthomolecular Medicine Today, April 26, 2016, Vancouver, ON. Reprinted with permission.

## Benefits of Low Dose Lithium

This book explores a vast collection of scientific literature on lithium in the areas of medicine, nutrition, biochemistry, psychiatry, and neurology. We have tried to help professionals, patients, and their families think outside the box and learn from decades of clinical experience in integrative medicine. We realize that this book involves a lot of information concerning the natural element lithium. The lithium dosages used in research exist from harmless drops to life-threatening pharmaceutical doses. Our goal is to improve the health of the millions suffering from neuropsychiatric impairments that are not responsive to traditional medical treatment models. Understanding the role of lithium is the key to unlocking brain health.

## CHAPTER 4 | References

Adams, J.B., Holloway, C.E., George, F., & Quig, D. (2006). Analyses of toxic metals and essential minerals in the hair of Arizona children with autism and associated conditions, and their mothers. *Biological Trace Element Research, 110*(3), 193-209.

Bagchi, N., Brown, T.R., & Mack R.E. (1978). Studies on the mechanism of inhibition of thyroid function by lithium. *Biochimia et Biophysica Acta, 542*(1), 163.

Druyan M.E., Bass, D., Puchyr, R, et al. (1998). Determination of reference ranges for elements in human scalp hair. *Biological Trace Element Research, 62*(3), 183-97.

Finley, P.R., Warner, M.D., & Peabody, C.A. (1995). Clinical relevance of drug interactions with lithium. *Clinical Pharmacokinetics, 29*(3), 172-191.

Kling, M. A., Manowitz, P., & Pollack, I. W. (1978). Rat brain and serum lithium concentrations after acute injections of lithium carbonate and orotate. *Journal of Pharmacy and Pharmacology, 30*(6), 368-370.

Kronemann, H., Anke, M., Groppel, B., Riedel, E. (1983). The capacity of organs to indicate the lithium level. In: Anke M, Baumann W, Bra¨unlich H, Bru¨ckner C (eds): *Proceedings 4. Spurenelement Symposium 1983*, Jena: VEB Kongressdruck, pp 85–93.

Li, X., Li, F., & Li, C.F. (2015). A new insight on the role of zinc in the regulation of altered thyroid functions during lithium treatment. Minerva Endocrinol. [Epub ahead of print]

Lieb, J. (1980). Linoleic acid in the treatment of lithium toxicity and familial tremor. *Prostaglandins Medicine, 4*(4), 257-9.

Manku, M. S., Horrobin, D. F., Karmazyn, M., & Cunnane, S. C. (1979). Prolactin and zinc effects on rat vascular reactivity: possible relationship to dihomo-gamma-linolenic acid and to prostaglandin synthesis. *Endocrinology, 104*(3), 774-779.

McKnight R.F., Adida, M., Budge, K., et al. (2012). Lithium toxicity profile: a systematic review and meta-analysis. *Lancet, 379*(9817), 721-8.

Mischley, L.K. (2012). *Lithium deficiency in Parkinson's Disease* (Doctoral dissertation). Retrieved from University of Washington.

Nieper, H. A. (1973). The clinical applications of lithium orotate. A two years study. *Agressologie, 14*(6), 407-411.

Pauze, D.K. & Brooks, D.E. (2007). Lithium toxicity from an internet dietary supplement. *Journal of Medical Toxicology, 3*(2), 61-2.

Sartori, H. E. (1986). Lithium orotate in the treatment of alcoholism and related conditions. *Alcohol, 3*(2), 97-100.

Schofer, J. & Schrauzer, G.N. (2011). Lithium and other elements in scalp hair of residents of Tokyo Prefecture as investigational predictors of suicide risk. *Biological Trace Element Research, 144*(1-3), 418-25.

Schrauzer, G.N. & de Vroey, E. (1994). Effects of nutritional lithium supplementation on mood. A placebo-controlled study with former drug users. *Biological Trace Element Research, 40*(1), 89-101.

Schrauzer, G.N. (2002). Lithium: occurrence, dietary intakes, nutritional essentiality. *Journal of the American College of Nutrition, 21*(1), 14-21.

Smith, D.F. & Schou, M. (1979). Kidney function and lithium concentrations of rats given an injection of lithium orotate or lithium carbonate. *Journal of Pharmacology and Pharmacotherapeutics, 31*(3), 161-3.

Watts, D. L. (1990). Nutrient interrelationships: minerals, vitamins, endocrines. *Journal of Orthomolecular Medicine, 5*(1), 11-19.

# Five

## LITHIUM AS A MINERAL: NEUROPROTECTION AND BRAIN HEALTH

Lithium is an essential nutrient for promoting brain health. Studies have shown clearly that the mineral lithium protects and stimulates the brain in complicated, multi-faceted ways—including cellular, molecular, and genetic influences. In this chapter we will explore the remarkable capabilities of this simple earth element to support the intricate inner function of the nervous system.

What starts as a small tube of tissue in the young embryo elegantly divides and folds to create the complex, multi-faceted human nervous system. The brain and knotted web of nerves that support it function instinctively at birth to help us to learn, create, explore, and navigate life on this planet. This blossoming of the nervous system from a simple cell to the sophisticated biochemical framework that houses our thoughts, emotions, and drive for survival is, quite simply, one of the great miracles of human life.

Traditionally, this phenomenon of nerve cell creation, called neurogenesis, was thought to occur exclusively in the early stages of life. After birth the brain increases in size four-fold during a child's preschool period, reaching approximately 90% of adult volume by age 6. After these very early stages, the growth of brain cells was believed to stop completely for the rest of the lifespan.

# Lithium as a Mineral: Neuroprotection and Brain Health

This classic image of the brain as a fixed, stagnant organ forecast a grave prognosis for anyone suffering from a neurological or psychiatric illness. Any malfunction in adult brain tissue was thought to be a permanent, devastating, and irreversible circumstance. This concept also led to a dismal outlook on aging, as brain cells are subject to wear and tear over time. Shrinking of the brain and loss of brain cells were painted as inevitable consequences of aging, just like graying hair or wrinkling skin.

Recent advances in technology and science, however, have shown that our earlier perception of the brain as possessing only a finite number of cells is not entirely accurate. While it is true that most neurons in the brain are generated before birth and never exchanged, new neurons and neural connections *can* be created in mammalian brains over the course of a lifetime. Neuronal synthesis is dependent on nutritional building blocks including amino acids, fatty acids, essential vitamins, and minerals such as lithium.

Here the role of lithium is reviewed as it pertains to the ongoing processes of neuroprotection, neurorepair and neurogenesis in the human brain.

## Lithium Enhances Neurotrophic Factors and Marker of Brain Cell Function

Neurotrophic factors are a group of proteins that regulate the growth and survival of neurons. The mineral lithium has been found to stimulate the circulation of several key neurotrophic factors, including brain-derived neurotrophic factor (BDNF) and neurotrophin-3 (NT-3) (Leyhe et al., 2009; Walz et al., 2008; Fukumoto et al., 2001).

### *LITHIUM PRIMES NEUROTROPHIC SYSTEM*

The BDNF protein is directly involved in the growth, maturation, and maintenance of nervous system cells. It is primarily found in the synapses, or spaces, between neurons, where it works to enhance cell-to-cell communication and signaling. Nerve cell synapses can strengthen and weaken over time in response to lived experience, a process of adaptation called synaptic plasticity.

BDNF also regulates this synaptic plasticity, an important biochemical underpinning of learning and memory preservation.

NT-3 is closely related to BDNF. As part of the Nerve Growth Factor family, it acts to promote the survival and differentiation of neurons in specific sections of the central nervous system. Most notably, NT-3 supports cellular resilience and helps to protect neurons from the harmful effects of stress and injury.

Not only does lithium increase circulating levels of these key proteins, but it also sensitizes the receptors that draw them into tissues. When the neurotrophic receptors are more alert, greater amounts of BDNF and NT-3 are drawn to help nervous system cells.

Lithium thus amplifies the effects of this brain-protecting neurotrophic system in two ways:

1. By increasing levels of neurotrophic factors, and
2. By allowing these proteins to work on cells more easily.

## *LITHIUM INCREASES MARKER OF NERVE CELL FUNCTION*

Other research has shown that lithium increases concentrations of a key chemical called N-acetyl-aspartate (NAA) in the human brain. NAA, one of the most concentrated molecules in the central nervous system, is crucial to nerve cell metabolism. It is therefore regarded as putative marker of neuronal integrity, with higher levels signifying increased brain cell function and viability (Moffett et al., 2007). At least 20 studies including a total of more than 300 child, adolescent, and adult subjects have explored brain metabolites such as NAA in neurological disease (Yilidiz & Ankerst, 2006). All studies have concluded that higher NAA counts are indeed predictive of better long-term cognitive function.

Several investigations have shown that lithium safely and effectively raises NAA concentrations in individuals of all ages. One cross-sectional assessment focused specifically on lithium treatment and NAA levels in older adults. Although the study sample was small, investigators found promising evidence that lithium could safely and effectively encourage healthy brain tissue development in elderly individuals (Forester et al., 2008).

# Lithium as a Mineral: Neuroprotection and Brain Health

| LITHIUM'S EFFECTS ON NEUROTROPHIC FACTORS AND MARKER OF BRAIN CELL FUNCTION |||
| --- | --- | --- |
| Lithium's Mechanisms | Role in the Brain | Implications For Brain Health |
| Increases the protein brain-derived neurotrophic factor (BDNF) | Regulates growth and survival of neurons | Supports growth and maintenance of nervous system cells, and enhances cell communication and signaling |
| Increases the protein neurotrophin-3 (NT-3) | Promotes survival and differentiation of neurons | Provides neurons protection from stress and injury |
| Increases the brain chemical N-acetyl-aspartate (NAA) | Serves a marker for neural viability | Enhances brain cell function and integrity |

## Lithium Balances Neurotransmitter Levels

Neurotransmitters are the chemical messengers that help to coordinate mood, appetite, sleep, movement and countless other biological processes. When levels of neurotransmitters are not balanced, dysfunctional behaviors follow. Maintaining an appropriate balance of these compounds is thus crucial to positive mental health. Lithium stabilizes the rate of neurotransmitter exchange in the brain, turning the activity up or down as needed.

### Lithium Optimizes Serotonin

Serotonin is one of the key neurotransmitters in the nervous system. It is biochemically synthesized from the amino acid tryptophan and is thought to be a primary contributor to feelings of well-being, satisfaction, and happiness.

From human studies we know that lithium has a net-enhancing effect on serotonin, meaning it optimizes the amount available for use in the brain and across other systems in the body (Chenu & Bourin, 2006; Bschor et al., 2002, 2003). Animal studies have provided a deeper understanding into how this occurs, and have shown that lithium works to support and balance the serotonergic system in a multitude of ways (Wegener et al., 2003). For example, lithium ions may repair problems with the synthesis, uptake, storage, release and/or catabolism of the neurotransmitter to ensure that there is an appropriate amount available to the cells. Some studies have even suggested that lithium improves the operation of the serotonin receptors as well (Price, 1990). Therefore, lithium does not simply increase or decrease serotonin levels, but helps to regulate its transport throughout the nervous system.

## *LITHIUM MODULATES DOPAMINE*

Dopamine is a dynamic neurotransmitter that works in many neurological pathways, including those for controlling locomotion, emotion, and cognition. Dopamine is most widely recognized for its role in the reward systems of the brain. Positive experiences, tasty foods, and addictive drugs trigger a rush of dopamine, leading to increased focus, motivation, and feelings of pleasure.

In order for this reward system to function properly, dopamine must be released in very precise, well-timed amounts. If too much dopamine floods the cells or if it stays in the synapse for an extended period of time, the surrounding cells can become agitated. Chronically elevated dopamine is implicated in a number of brain-based disorders including schizophrenia and affective disorders. Lithium salts have been shown in multiple studies to counteract dopamine-induced hyperactivity and to restore proper dopamine transport. The exact mechanism of lithium's dopamine-antagonizing effects are unclear, although there is some research to show that lithium ions alter the sensitivity of dopamine receptors to reduce excitatory effects (Beaulieu et al., 2004; Del' Guidice & Beaulieu, 2015).

Other studies have found that lithium salts can increase dopamine when levels are too low. In Parkinson's disease, declining dopamine concentrations result in motor abnormalities. One study in Parkinson's patients found that low doses of lithium boosted the expression of tyrosine hydroxylase, an enzyme that increases dopamine synthesis (Lazzara et al., 2015). These complementary results highlight the fact that the actions of lithium are not simple and unidirectional, but rather dependent on a number of circumstantial factors and highly responsive to neurophysiological conditions in the brain.

## *LITHIUM REGULATES GLUTAMATE*

Glutamate is the major excitatory neurotransmitter in the brain. Under healthy physiological conditions it promotes the biological processes involved with learning and memory, and also aids in high-level cognitive integration. However, in some neurological disorders the production of this neurotransmitter increases and its clearance from synapses slows. This combination leads to an excess of glutamate in brain tissue that over-stimulates the cells. Under these hyper-excitable conditions, neurons become agitated and injured, eventually causing cell death (Hamilton, Zamponi & Ferguson, 2015).

Lithium works by deactivating N-methyl-D-aspartate (NMDA) receptors, the main class of glutamate receptors in the nervous tissue. By preventing the uptake of glutamate, lithium thus buffers the cells against its damaging, excitotoxic effects. Remarkably, lithium exerts these neuroprotective capabilities when used at doses below those considered "therapeutic" in mainstream medicine (Hashimoto et al., 2002). The regulation of intracellular glutamate levels is another pathway through which lithium provides equilibrium in the nervous system and stabilizes mood.

### *Lithium Modulates Monoamine Oxidase Activity*

Monoamine oxidase (MAO) is an enzyme that breaks down certain neurotransmitters in the body including norepinephrine, dopamine, and serotonin. Levels of MAO determine how much of a neurotransmitter is available to neurons at any given time. In a healthy nervous system, monoamine oxidase activity is highly regulated to maintain balanced neurotransmitter levels and a favorable mental state.

When MAO activity decreases, neurotransmitters are not broken down appropriately, and an overabundance can be left in the nervous system. This is often the case in chronic aggression and the manic phase of bipolar disorder, wherein elevated dopamine and norepinephrine drive impulsive, sensation-seeking behaviors. Lower MAO A activity has been associated with increased severity and frequency of impulsive, violent, or abusive behaviors as well (Alia-Klein et al., 2008).

In these situations, lithium stabilizes monoamine oxidase activity by increasing its ability to break down excitatory neurotransmitters. Interestingly, there is also evidence to show that lithium can reduce monoamine oxidase activity (Fisar, Hroudova & Raboch, 2010). This inhibitory action would prove more useful in conditions such as depression, where lower neurotransmitter levels may be the central issue. These complementary actions suggest that lithium has adaptogenic actions on the monoamine oxidase system. Lithium can calibrate enzyme activity in either direction, depending on what may be required to maintain homeostasis.

| LITHIUM'S EFFECTS ON NEUROTRANSMITTER BALANCE |||
| --- | --- | --- |
| Lithium's Mechanisms | Role in the Brain | Implications For Brain Health |
| Increases neurotransmitter serotonin | Regulation of mood, behavior, appetite, and memory | Increase in serotonin bioavailability is able to correct abnormalities involved in pathogenesis of mood disorders |
| Increases neurotransmitter dopamine | Regulation of locomotion, emotion, cognition, and reward systems | Alleviates mood swings and excitability |
| Decreases excitatory neurotransmitter glutamate | Involved in cellular metabolism and neural activation; aids in learning and memory | Reduces hyper-excitatory conditions that result in damaged neurons |
| Increases the enzymatic action of monoamine oxidase | Breakdown of neurotransmitters including norepinephrine, dopamine, and serotonin | Provides balance between multiple neurotransmitter systems; reduces chronic aggression resulting from insufficient MAO activity |

## Lithium Decreases Inflammation

Neuroinflammation is the inflammation of nervous tissue. Normally, this is a protective process coordinated by the immune system and occurring in response to an irritating trigger such as infection, toxic metabolites, or traumatic injury. Inflammation is meant to stimulate repair and recovery in brain tissue by delivering white blood cells and other healing constituents. However, if not controlled properly, this process can be very damaging.

### LITHIUM SUPPRESSES PRO-INFLAMMATORY CYTOKINES

Scientists now believe that a key component in many chronic mental health disorders is rampant, wide-spread neuroinflammation. In disorders as diverse as depression and Alzheimer's disease, researchers have found that the inflammatory response becomes disrupted and proceeds in an out-of-control manner (Moore & O'Banion, 2002). Control over this process is predicted to be a key clinical target for arresting neuron destruction and stabilizing brain health. Cells in the immune system communicate by releasing and responding to chemical messengers known as cytokines. Cytokines include a diverse assortment of interleukins, interferons, and growth factors. Lithium helps to moderate inflammation by dampening cytokine reactivity. In particular, it reduces the production of two pro-inflammatory cytokines known as interleukin-1B and tumor necrosis factor. Lithium also suppresses the resident immune cells in the brain and spinal cord, called the microglia, so that they do not become over-stimulated (Nahman et al., 2012).

### *Lithium Changes Fatty Acid Expression*
Chronic lithium therapy changes fatty acid metabolism in the brain in a way that protects against inflammation. The release of arachidonic acid, an unstable and reactive polyunsaturated omega-6 fatty acid, is blocked. Meanwhile, the formation of the reparative docosahexaenoic omega-3 fatty acid, also called DHA, is bolstered (Basselin et al., 2010). By shifting these factors at various points in the inflammatory chain, lithium significantly diminishes neuroinflammation, protecting neurons from devastating effects.

| LITHIUM REDUCES INFLAMMATION |||
| --- | --- | --- |
| Lithium's Mechanisms | Role in the Brain | Implications For Brain Health |
| Suppresses pro-inflammatory cytokines | Chemical messengers of the immune system; if unregulated cause cell death | Reduces oxidative damage caused by pro-inflammatory cytokines |
| Inhibits release of arachidonic acid | Mediates inflammatory reactions | Exerts anti-inflammatory effects by increasing levels of the fish oil compound DHA (docosahexaenoic acid) |

## Lithium Provides Metabolic Support
The mineral lithium is absorbed as a salt via channels in the small intestines. It is then distributed ubiquitously throughout body water and deposited in bone and hair (Mischley, 2012). Along the way, lithium ions interact with other nutrients to complete several key metabolic tasks.

# Nutritional Lithium: A Cinderella Story

*LITHIUM HELPS WITH B12 AND FOLATE TRANSPORT*
Lithium is necessary for the transport of vitamin B12 and folate into cells (Schopfer & Schrauzer, 2011). Depressed patients on pharmacologic doses of lithium have been shown to have higher levels of serum B12 and folic acid than controls (Tisman, Herbert & Rosenblatt, 1973; Abou-Sale & Coppen, 1989). These vitamins have significant effects on the central nervous system and work in collaboration to support many biochemical processes critical to bolstering mood and stabilizing behavior. Vitamin B12, for example, is required for coating nerve cells in myelin- a fatty, protective substance that enhances communication between nerve cells. Folate works to promote accurate nerve cell signaling by increasing the production of S-adenosylmethionine, or SAM-e, a compound that is used in the synthesis of neurotransmitters.

Lithium plays a role in supporting healthy intercellular communication in the nervous system by facilitating vitamin B12 and folate transport across cell membranes. Increasing vitamin B12 and folate transport is a basic pathway through which lithium regulates mood and behavior (Schrauzer, Shrestha & Flores-Acre, 1992).

*LITHIUM PROTECTS AGAINST FREE RADICALS*
Oxidative stress is a state that occurs when there is an imbalance between the presence of damaging molecules known as free radicals and the ability of the body to counteract their harmful effects with antioxidants. Free radicals readily and negatively alter the lipids, proteins, and DNA that make up brain cells, triggering disease processes in the nervous system. Researchers speculate that cellular oxidation often occurs in the human brain as a result of cumulative, long-term exposures to free radicals in the environment. This could include contact with toxic chemicals, physical injury, or chronic stress.

Lithium ions work to curb free radical forces by increasing antioxidant defenses in the peripheral and central nervous system (Andreazza et al., 2008). Primarily, lithium increases levels of glutathione in the brain (Cui et al., 2007). Glutathione is an antioxidant naturally found within every cell in the body. While many vitamins, minerals, and phytochemicals also act as antioxidants,

# Lithium as a Mineral: Neuroprotection and Brain Health

glutathione is unique because it is intracellular and produced inherently. Adequate glutathione levels are actually required so that other antioxidants such as vitamins C, E, selenium, and carotenoids, can be properly utilized.

By bolstering production of glutathione, the "master antioxidant," lithium reinforces the entire antioxidant network in cells. Lithium therapy thereby protects the nervous system against aggregate damage from oxidative stress.

## *Lithium Improves Mitochondrial Function*

Most diseases of the brain coincide with a reduction in neuron metabolism. This effect is often attributed to a malfunction in the mitochondria— the organelles that generate energy for cells. As the "power houses" of the cell, mitochondria are involved in a wide range of basic functions, including metabolism, signaling cell differentiation, and cell death. Needless to say, these small structures are vital to the maintenance of healthy cells and tissues.

Mitochondrial defects are observed in a striking number of health conditions, including neurodegenerative diseases, aging, and cancer. Recognition of this connection has made the mitochondria a focus area for the development of early detection and treatment strategies (Dimauro & Davidzon, 2005). Recent work with bipolar patients has demonstrated that lithium increases mitochondrial mass and the ability of these organelles to generate energy for the cells (Struewing et al., 2007; Forester et al., 2008). For dementia sufferers and others struggling with neurological disease, the mitochondrial support provided by lithium can help reignite failing brain tissue metabolism.

| LITHIUM PROVIDES METABOLIC SUPPORT |||
|---|---|---|
| **Lithium's Mechanisms** | **Role in the Brain** | **Implications For Brain Health** |
| Assists in vitamin $B_{12}$ and folate transport | Important cofactors involved in the synthesis of serotonin and dopamine | Increase in energy; decreases in mood swings, depression, irritability, dementia, and mania symptoms |
| Reduces free radicals | Oxidative stress that triggers disease processes by disrupting lipids, proteins, and DNA structures | Produces the antioxidant glutathione to protect against oxidative stress |
| Boosts mitochondrial function | Generates energy for cells; responsible for regulating metabolism and signaling cell differentiation and cell death | Increases mitochondrial mass and ability to generate energy for cells |

## Lithium Increases Neuronal Integrity
Neurons exist in a dynamic equilibrium that is constantly influenced by extracellular physiological changes. Lithium has the ability to balance intracellular responses, thereby increasing the strength and resilience of nervous system cells.

### *Lithium Inhibits Brain Damaging Enzyme*
Lithium regulates an enzyme known as Glycogen Synthase Kinase-3 (GSK3). This unique enzyme modifies over forty different proteins throughout the body, making it crucial for a wide range of biological processes. GKS-3 is known to support a wide range of biological functions ranging from glucose metabolism to gene transcription (Jope & Roh, 2006). In the nervous system, GSK3 plays a major role in neural growth and development. It works to regulate insulin transport and immune response to nourish and protect the brain cells. Notably, specific levels of GSK3 are required to carry out the process of synaptic remodeling, which drives memory formation (Hooper, Killick & Loves, 2008). GSK3 activity must be tightly regulated to maintain healthy signaling pathways in mature brain tissue.

In certain neuropsychiatric illnesses, however, GSK3 becomes sporadically hyperactive. This up-regulation spurs the enzyme to phosphorylate, or activate, proteins in the nerve cells at an aberrantly high rate. Among GSK3s target proteins are amyloid-B and tau proteins, which rapidly accumulate to create blockages in the brain tissue. Local inflammatory and immune cascades are also triggered, resulting in widespread neuronal damage.

Lithium is a GSK3 inhibitor. By preventing the over-expression of GKS-3, lithium helps to stop inappropriate protein production and activation (Hooper, Killick & Loves, 2008; Wada, 2009; Engel et al., 2006).

### *Lithium "Cleans" Plaques and Tangles*
All cells have a built-in cleaning system that breaks down and discards unnecessary or dysfunctional cell components. This is called autophagy. Autophagic processes are important for balancing energy and clearing out stores of abnormal, mutant, or disease-prone proteins. However, in many neuropsychiatric and neurodegenerative illnesses, autophagy is disabled. With autophagic

systems disarmed, dysfunctional proteins and toxins can accumulate much faster and with more deleterious effects to brain tissue (Cheung & Ip, 2011).

Lithium treatment has been shown to stimulate autophagy. Lithium activates the mechanism for discarding cellular waste by inhibiting an enzyme known as inositol monophosphatase (IMPase). Normally, IMPase works to promote the recycling of important signaling molecules in the cells (Harwood, 2005). When lithium blocks IMPase, this recycling system stops, and autophagic process are used to clean up any incomplete or damaged molecules that may be leftover in the cells.

Lithium's ability to increase autophagy is highly useful for removing unwanted amyloid beta and tau proteins. By encouraging the cells to "clean-up" using their own intrinsic waste removal system, lithium supports the removal of restrictive proteins without harm to the healthy tissues (Sarkar, et al., 2005; Ravikumar, et al., 2010).

## *Lithium Helps Healthy Cells Survive*

For cells that are too damaged to be cleaned out and rejuvenated through autophagy, calculated cell destruction is necessary. Apoptosis is the routine process of programmed cell death that clears unneeded cells from the body. In some neurological diseases apoptosis becomes dysregulated, however, and perfectly healthy cells are destroyed, contributing to neuron loss (Shimohama, 2000).

Normally, the process of apoptosis is governed by two opposing groups of molecules. Anti-apoptotic molecules are present in healthy cells and serve to signal when cell death is not necessary. Molecules in this group include compounds called B-cell lymphoma-2 (bcl-2) and B-catenin. The other group is made-up of pro-apoptotic molecules that flag cells as damaged and indicate that they should be removed. Molecules in the pro-apoptotic group include tumor protein p53, Bcl-2-associated X protein (Bax), and caspases (Liechti et al., 2014). Both groups of molecules must be present in an intricate balance to ensure that healthy cells survive, while injured or unwanted cells are removed from the body (Manji, 1999; Chen et al., 1999).

Lithium helps to maintain even and appropriate levels of both groups of apoptotic molecules. In the face of neurodegenerative diseases like Alzheimer's, this means up-regulating molecules that prevent apoptosis and turning down the expression of those that support it for a net effect of slowing down cell death.

By adjusting the rate of apoptosis, or cell death, in the tissues, lithium thus holds a remarkable potential to stop the unchecked tissue loss that is characteristic of many psychiatric and neurodegenerative diseases.

| LITHIUM SUPPORTS NEURONAL INTEGRITY ||| 
|---|---|---|
| **Lithium's Mechanisms** | **Role in the Brain** | **Implications For Brain Health** |
| Inhibits the enzyme glycogen synthase kinase 3 (GSK3) | Supports biological functions including gene transcription, insulin transport, and immune response | Inhibits inappropriate amyloid production and hyper-phosphorylation of tau proteins |
| Stimulates autophagy | Instrinsic waste system that discards dysfunctional cell components | Autophagic process removes damaged molecules of amyloid beta and tau proteins without harming healthy tissues |
| Regulates apoptosis | Programmed cell death to remove cellular waste | Maintains balance of apoptotic molecules without harming healthy neurons |

## Lithium Supports Neurogenesis

Neurogenesis is the process of nerve cell creation, often called the "birth of new neurons." Neuron formation occurs most rapidly during the early years of human growth and development, but it can continue on at a slower pace later in life when key physiological and nutritional factors are present.

### *Lithium Increases Gray Matter*

Studies using Magnetic Resonance Imaging (MRI) techniques to scan the brain provided the first hard evidence of lithium's beneficial and growth-promoting effects. In one early project, researchers looked at the brain volume in 12 bipolar patients who were taking lithium to regulate mood (Sassi et al., 2002). The team was shocked by what they found when they reviewed the MRI images: patients taking lithium had a significantly larger amount of total gray matter—the brain tissue containing brain cell bodies—compared to other bipolar patients who were not taking lithium. The patients on lithium had more gray matter than healthy controls.

# Lithium as a Mineral: Neuroprotection and Brain Health

A similar study focused specifically on lithium's effects on the hippocampus, a small region of the brain involved in emotion and memory (Bearden et al., 2008). The results were surprisingly similar: the hippocampal volume was 14% higher in the lithium-treated patients than in bipolar patients taking no medication, and 10% higher than the levels found in healthy controls. At least three other studies of varying design have replicated these results, suggesting that lithium has remarkable stimulating effects on brain growth and repair (Kempton et al., 2008).

### *LITHIUM ENHANCES NERVE CELL GROWTH*

Of all research reviewing lithium's neurotrophic effects, the most captivating proof came from a study that assessed what happened when an isolated nerve cell was bathed in a lithium solution. Remarkably, this lone cell began to regenerate and grow when exposed to lithium. Dramatic changes were seen particularly in the number and length of the dendrites of the neuron—the antennae-like structures that branch out from the main cell and serve as the primary apparatus for receiving signals from other nerve cells (Dwivedi & Zhang, 2014). Other studies have revealed that tissues exposed to lithium show a striking increase in the proliferation of progenitor cells, the stem-cell like precursor cells that rapidly divide to create new tissues (Hashimoto et al., 2003; Kim et al., 2004).

| LITHIUM ENHANCES NEUROGENESIS ||| 
| --- | --- | --- |
| **Lithium's Mechanisms** | **Role in the Brain** | **Implications For Brain Health** |
| Increases gray matter in the brain | Route sensory or motor stimuli to neurons that transmit and process information throughout the CNS | Prevention or partial reversal of regional gray matter deficits |
| Regenerates nerve cells and increases length of dendrites | Transmission of messages | Enhances cell-to-cell communication |

## Protecting the Brain with Lithium

Scientists used to think that the human brain reached a developmental standstill with the advent of adulthood. It was considered scientific dogma that the brain and nervous system had a finite number of cells, and that any damage to neurons was permanent and irreversible. It is now recognized, however, that under the right conditions, the brain holds the potential to create new neurons and neural connections throughout the lifespan.

Lithium has distinct and often dramatic neurotrophic effects, encouraging the survival and growth of nerve cells. Lithium ions modulate multiple biological cascades involved with nerve cell development. Lithium increases levels of key proteins such as BDNF and NT-3, which are known to be directly involved in nerve cell development. Other studies have found that lithium salts are neuroprotective, working to minimize inflammation, enhance mitochondrial function, and increase antioxidants to provide the optimal environment for neurons to thrive. Imaging studies have provided visual evidence that patients taking lithium salts experience increases in brain tissue volume over time, particularly in the gray matter of the brain, which holds the nerve cell bodies. At the cellular level lithium exerts powerful influences on neuroprotection and brain health. In the next chapter we will look at how this mineral may also help to optimize the expression of our genes for long-term neurological health.

# Lithium as a Mineral: Neuroprotection and Brain Health

| LITHIUM'S MECHANISMS | ROLE IN THE BRAIN | IMPLICATIONS FOR BRAIN HEALTH |
|---|---|---|
| *NEUROTROPHIC FACTORS AND BIOMARKER FOR BRAIN FUNCTION* | | |
| Increases the protein brain-derived neurotrophic factor (BDNF) | Regulates growth and survival of neurons | Supports growth and maintenance of nervous system cells, and enhances cell communication and signaling |
| Increases the protein neurotrophin-3 (NT-3) | Promotes survival and differentiation of neurons | Provides neurons protection from stress and injury |
| Increases the brain chemical N-acetyl-aspartate (NAA) | Serves a marker for neural viability | Enhances brain cell function and integrity |
| *NEUROTRANSMITTER BALANCE* | | |
| Increases neurotransmitter serotonin | Regulation of mood, behavior, appetite, and memory | Increase in serotonin bioavailability is able to correct abnormalities involved in pathogenesis of mood disorders |
| Increases neurotransmitter dopamine | Regulation of locomotion, emotion, cognition, and reward systems | Alleviates mood swings and excitability |
| Decreases excitatory neurotransmitter glutamate | Involved in cellular metabolism and neural activation; aids in learning and memory | Reduces hyper-excitatory conditions that result in damaged neurons |
| Increases the enzymatic action of monoamine oxidase | Breakdown of neurotransmitters including norepinephrine, dopamine, and serotonin | Provides balance between multiple neurotransmitter systems; reduces chronic aggression resulting from insufficient MAO activity |
| *INFLAMMATION* | | |
| Suppresses pro-inflammatory cytokines | Chemical messengers of the immune system; if unregulated cause cell death | Reduces oxidative damage caused by pro-inflammatory cytokines |
| Inhibits release of arachidonic acid | Mediates inflammatory reactions | Exerts anti-inflammatory effects by increasing levels of the fish oil compound DHA (docosahexaenoic acid) |

# Nutritional Lithium: A Cinderella Story

| LITHIUM'S MECHANISMS | ROLE IN THE BRAIN | IMPLICATIONS FOR BRAIN HEALTH |
|---|---|---|
| *METABOLIC SUPPORT* | | |
| Assists in vitamin $B_{12}$/ folate transport | Important cofactors involved in the synthesis of serotonin and dopamine | Increase in energy; decreases in mood swings, depression, irritability, dementia, and mania symptoms |
| Reduces free radicals | Oxidative stress that triggers disease processes by disrupting lipids, proteins, and DNA structures | Produces the antioxidant glutathione to protect against oxidative stress |
| Boosts mitochondrial function | Generates energy for cells; responsible for regulating metabolism and signaling cell differentiation and cell death | Increases mitochondrial mass and ability to generate energy for cells |
| *NEURONAL INTEGRITY* | | |
| Inhibits the enzyme glycogen synthase kinase 3 (GSK3) | Supports biological functions including gene transcription, insulin transport, and immune response | Inhibits inappropriate amyloid production and hyper-phosphorylation of tau proteins |
| Stimulates autophagy | Instrinsic waste system that discards dysfunctional cell components | Autophagic process removes damaged molecules of amyloid beta and tau proteins without harming healthy tissues |
| Regulates apoptosis | Programmed cell death to remove cellular waste | Maintains balance of apoptotic molecules without harming healthy neurons |
| *NEUROGENESIS* | | |
| Increases gray matter in the brain | Route sensory or motor stimuli to neurons that transmit and process information throughout the CNS | Prevention or partial reversal of regional gray matter deficits |
| Regenerates nerve cells and increases length of dendrites | Transmission of messages | Enhances cell-to-cell communication |

*Figures 5.1 to 5.2 Summary of lithium's proposed mechanisms in providing neuroprotection and promoting brain health.*

## CHAPTER 5 | References

Abou-Saleh, M. T., & Coppen, A. (1989). Serum and red blood cell folate in depression. *Acta Psychiatrica Scandinavica, 80*(1), 78-82.

Alia-Klein, N., Goldstein, R. Z., Kriplani, A., Logan, J., Tomasi, D., Williams, B., & ... Fowler, J. S. (2008). Brain monoamine oxidase A activity predicts trait aggression. *The Journal Of Neuroscience, 28*(19), 5099-5104.

Andreazza, A. C., Anna, M. K., Frey, B. N., et al. (2008). Oxidative stress markers in bipolar disorder: A meta-analysis. *Journal of Affective Disorders, 111*(2-3), 135-144.

Basselin, M., Kim, H., Chen, M., Ma, K., Rapoport, S. I., Murphy, R. C., & Farias, S. E. (2010). Lithium modifies brain arachidonic and docosahexaenoic metabolism in rat lipopolysaccharide model of neuroinflammation. *Journal of Lipid Research, 51*(5), 1049-1056.

Bearden, C. E., Thompson, P. M., Dutton, R. A., et al. (2008). Three-dimensional mapping of hippocampal anatomy in unmedicated and lithium-treated patients with bipolar disorder. *Neuropsychopharmacology, 33*(6), 1229-1238.

Beaulieu, J., Sotnikova, T. D., Yao, W., et al. (2004). Lithium antagonizes dopamine-dependent behaviors mediated by an AKT/glycogen synthase kinase cascade. *Proceedings of the National Academy of Sciences of the United States of America, 101*(14), 5099-104.

Bschor, T., Adli, M., Baethge, C., Eichmann, U., Ising, M., Uhr, M., & ... Bauer, M. (2002). Lithium augmentation increases the ACTH and cortisol response in the combined DEX/CRH test in unipolar major depression. *Neuropsychopharmacology, 27*(3), 470-478.

Bschor, T., Baethge, C., Adli, M., Eichmann, U., Ising, M., Uhr, M., & ... Bauer, M. (2003). Association between response to lithium augmentation and the combined DEX/CRH test in major depressive disorder. *Journal of Psychiatric Research, 37*(2), 135-143.

Chen, G., Zeng, W. Z., Yuan, P. X., Huang, L. D., Jiang, Y. M., Zhao, Z. H., & Manji, H. K. (1999). The mood-stabilizing agents lithium and valproate robustly increase the levels of the neuroprotective protein bcl-2 in the CNS. *Journal of Neurochemistry, 72*(2), 879-882.

Chenu, F., & Bourin, M. (2006). Potentiation of antidepressant-like activity with lithium: mechanism involved. *Current Drug Targets, 7*(2), 159-163.

Cheung, Z. H., & Ip, N. Y. (2011). Autophagy deregulation in neurodegenerative diseases - recent advances and future perspectives. *Journal of Neurochemistry, 118*(3), 317.

Cui, J., Shao, L., Young, L., & Wang, J. (2007). Role of glutathione in neuroprotective effects of mood stabilizing drugs lithium and valproate. *Neuroscience, 144*(4), 1447-53.

Del' Guidice, T., & Beaulieu, J. (2015). Selective disruption of dopamine D2-receptors/beta-arrestin2 signaling by mood stabilizers. *Journal of Receptor and Signal Transduction Research, 35*(3), 224-232.

Dimauro, S., & Davidzon, G. (2005). Mitochondrial DNA and disease. *Annals of Medicine, 37*(3), 222-232.

Dwivedi, T., & Zhang, H. (2015). Lithium-induced neuroprotection is associated with epigenetic modification of specific BDNF gene promoter and altered expression of apoptotic-regulatory proteins. *Frontiers in Neuroscience, 8*, 457.

Engel, T., Goni-Oliver, P., Lucas, J. J., Avila, J., & Hernandez, F. (2006). Chronic lithium administration to FTDP-17 tau and GSK-3beta overexpressing mice prevents tau hyperphosphorylation and neurofibrillary tangle formation, but pre-formed neurofibrillary tangles do not revert. *Journal of Neurochemistry, 99*(6), 1445-55.

Fisar, Z., Hroudová, J., & Raboch, J. (2010). Inhibition of monoamine oxidase activity by antidepressants and mood stabilizers. *Neuro Endocrinology Letters, 31*(5), 645-656.

Forester, B. P., Finn, C. T., Berlow, Y. A., Wardrop, M., Renshaw, P. F., & Moore, C. M. (2008). Brain lithium, N-acetyl aspartate and myo-inositol levels in older adults with bipolar disorder treated with lithium: a lithium-7 and proton magnetic resonance spectroscopy study. *Bipolar Disorders, 10*(6), 691-700.

Fukumoto, T., Morinobu, S., Okamoto, Y., Kagaya, A., & Yamawaki, S. (2001). Chronic lithium treatment increases the expression of brain-derived neurotrophic factor in the rat brain. *Psychopharmacology, 158*(1), 100-106.

Hamilton, A., Zamponi, G. W., & Ferguson, S. G. (2015). Glutamate receptors function as scaffolds for the regulation of β-amyloid and cellular prion protein signaling complexes. *Molecular Brain, 8*, 18.

Harwood, A. J. (2005). Lithium and bipolar mood disorder: The inositol-depletion hypothesis revisited. *Molecular Psychiatry, 10*(1), 117-126.

Hashimoto, R., Hough, C., Nakazawa, T., Yamamoto, T., & Chuang, D. (2002). Lithium protection against glutamate excitotoxicity in rat cerebral cortical neurons: involvement of NMDA receptor inhibition possibly by decreasing NR2B tyrosine phosphorylation. *Journal of Neurochemistry, 80*(4), 589-597.

Hashimoto, R., Senatorov, V., Kanai, H., Leeds, P., & Chuang, D. (2003). Lithium stimulates progenitor proliferation in cultured brain neurons. *Neuroscience, 117*(1), 55-61.

Hooper, C., Killick, R., & Lovestone, S. (2008). The GSK3 hypothesis of Alzheimer's disease. *Journal of Neurochemistry, 104*(6), 1433.

Jope, R. S., & Roh, M. (2006). Glycogen synthase kinase-3 (GSK3) in psychiatric diseases and therapeutic interventions. *Current Drug Targets, 7*(11), 1421-1434.

Kempton, M. J., Geddes, J. R., Ettinger, U., Williams, S. C., & Grasby, P. M. (2008). Meta-analysis, database, and meta-regression of 98 structural imaging studies in bipolar disorder. *Archives of General Psychiatry, 65*(9), 1017-32.

Kim, J. S., Chang, M., Yu, I. T., Kim, J. H., Lee, S., Lee, Y., & Son, H. (2004). Lithium selectively increases neuronal differentiation of hippocampal neural progenitor cells both in vitro and in vivo. *Journal of Neurochemistry, 89*(2), 324-336.

Lazzara, C. A., Riley, R. R., Rane, A., Andersen, J. K., & Kim, Y. (2015). The combination of lithium and l-Dopa/Carbidopa reduces MPTP-induced abnormal involuntary movements (AIMs) via calpain-1 inhibition in a mouse model: Relevance for Parkinson's disease therapy. *Brain Research, 1622*, 127-136.

Liechti, F. D., Stüdle, N., Theurillat, R., Grandgirard, D., Thormann, W., & Leib, S. L. (2014). The mood-stabilizer lithium prevents hippocampal apoptosis and improves spatial memory in experimental meningitis. *Plos One, 9*(11), e113607.

Leyhe, T., Eschweiler, G. W., Stransky, E., Gasser, T., Annas, P., Basun, H., & Laske, C. (2009). Increase of BDNF serum concentration in lithium treated patients with early Alzheimer's disease. *Journal Of Alzheimer's Disease, 16*(3), 649-656.

Manji, H. K., Moore, G. J., & Chen, G. (1999). Lithium at 50: Have the neuroprotective effects of this unique cation been overlooked? *Biological Psychiatry, 46*(7), 929-940.

Mischley, L. (2012). Lithium deficiency in Parkinson's disease. University of Washington MPH thesis. Unpublished.

Moffett, J. R., Ross, B., Arun, P., Madhavarao, C. N., & Namboodiri, A. M. (2007). N- Acetylaspartate in the CNS: From neurodiagnostics to neurobiology. *Progress in Neurobiology, 81*(2), 89-131.

Moore, A. H., & O'Banion, M. (2002). Neuroinflammation and antiinflammatory therapy for Alzheimer's disease. *Advanced Drug Delivery Reviews, 54*(12):1627-56.

Nahman, S., Belmaker, R. H., & Azab, A. N. (2012). Effects of lithium on lipopolysaccharide-induced inflammation in rat primary glia cells. *Innate Immunity, 18*(3), 447-458.

Price, L. H., Charney, D. S., Delgado, P. L., & Heninger, G. R. (1990). Lithium and serotonin function: Implications for the serotonin hypothesis of depression. *Psychopharmacology, 100*(1), 3-12.

Ravikumar, B., Sarkar, S., Davies, J. E., Futter, M., Garcia-Arencibia, M., Green-Thompson, Z. W., & ... Rubinsztein, D. C. (2010). Regulation of mammalian autophagy in physiology and pathophysiology. *Physiological Reviews, 90*(4), 1383-435.

Sarkar, S., Floto, R. A., Berger, Z., Imarisio, S., Cordenier, A., Pasco, M., & ... Rubinsztein, D. C. (2005). Lithium Induces Autophagy by Inhibiting Inositol Monophosphatase. *The Journal of Cell Biology, 170*(7), 1101-11.

Sassi, R. B., Nicoletti, M., Brambilla, P., Mallinger, A. G., Frank, E., Kupfer, D. J., & ... Soares, J. C. (2002). Increased gray matter volume in lithium-treated bipolar disorder patients. *Neuroscience Letters, 329*(2), 243-245.

Schrauzer, G. N., Shrestha, K. P., & Flores-Arce, M. F. (1992). Lithium in scalp hair of adults, students, and violent criminals. Effects of supplementation and evidence for interactions of lithium with vitamin B12 and with other trace elements. *Biological Trace Element Research, 34*(2), 161-176.

Schöpfer, J., & Schrauzer, G. N. (2011). Lithium and other elements in scalp hair of residents of Tokyo Prefecture as investigational predictors of suicide risk. *Biological Trace Element Research, 144*(1-3), 418-425.

Shimohama, S. (2000). Apoptosis in Alzheimer's disease—an update. *Apoptosis, 5*(1), 9-16.

Struewing, I. T., Barnett, C. D., Tang, T., & Mao, C. D. (2007). Lithium increases PGC-1alpha expression and mitochondrial biogenesis in primary bovine aortic endothelial cells. *FEBS Journal, 274*(11), 2749.

Tisman, G., Herbert, V., & Rosenblatt, S. (1973). Evidence that Lithium Induces Human Granulocyte Proliferation: Elevated Serum Vitamin B12 Binding Capacity in Vivo and Granulocyte Colony Proliferation in Vitro. *British Journal of Haematology, 24*(6), 767.

Wada, A. (2009). Lithium and neuropsychiatric therapeutics: neuroplasticity via glycogen synthase kinase-3beta, beta-catenin, and neurotrophin cascades. *Journal of Pharmacological Sciences, 110*(1), 14-28.

Walz, J. C., Frey, B. N., Andreazza, A. C., Cereśer, K. M., Cacilhas, A. A., Valvassori, S. S., & ... Kapczinski, F. (2008). Effects of lithium and valproate on serum and hippocampal neurotrophin-3 levels in an animal model of mania. *Journal of Psychiatric Research, 42*(5), 416-421.

Wegener, G., Bandpey, Z., Heiberg, I. L., Mørk, A., & Rosenberg, R. (2003). Increased extracellular serotonin level in rat hippocampus induced by chronic citalopram is augmented by subchronic lithium: Neurochemical and behavioural studies in the rat. *Psychopharmacology, 166*(2), 188-194.

Yildiz-Yesiloglu, A., & Ankerst, D. P. (2006). Neurochemical alterations of the brain in bipolar disorder and their implications for pathophysiology: A systematic review of the in vivo proton magnetic resonance spectroscopy findings. *Progress in Neuropsychopharmacology & Biological Psychiatry, 30*(6), 969-95.

# Six

## LITHIUM AS A MINERAL: ORCHESTRATING OUR GENES

Lithium's dramatic effects on the brain go beyond changes at the cellular level. We now know that lithium can even change the way genes are expressed. These new discoveries come from recent research at the frontier of science and medicine. They will likely redefine the prevention and treatment of psychiatric and neurological illness.

Already, scientists have upended our former understanding of genetics. Ever since Gregory Mendel's research, genetic heritage was considered fixed at birth, in contrast to the environmental forces that influence individuals as they grow. "Nature" and "nurture" were conceptualized as opposing forces. We now realize that the influence of genetics on health is much more complicated than just the DNA sequence in an individual's genes. The idea of a dichotomy between unchanging nature and variable nurture has been replaced by a newer understanding based on science: our genetic code is more changeable than we knew. Although genes themselves may not change, whether and how much a gene is expressed are infinitely variable.

The earliest striking evidence of changes in gene expression involves people born during and just after the Dutch Hunger Winter, the winter of 1944-1945. During this last winter of the Second World War, the Germans set up a blockade to keep food and fuel from reaching the western part of the Netherlands. Consequently, many of the Dutch in this area experienced a severe shortage of food. Some people were limited to as few as 500 calories a day during that winter (Tobi et al., 2014).

Fifty years later, a clear pattern emerged. Those now middle-aged people who were conceived when food was most scarce weighed an average of 14 pounds more, had an average waist size 1 ½ inches larger, and were three times more likely to suffer from heart disease than those whose mothers were in the second or third trimester during the Dutch Hunger Winter. Researchers found that an important gene for growth was more expressed, or turned on, in people conceived during the worst of the period of starvation. Those born just six months later had less expression of this growth gene. These results were the first evidence that environmental conditions of life even in utero can cause changes that persist through life. The changes altered the fetuses' metabolism so they could get the most from the scant nutrients they received. Because this "thrifty metabolism" never reversed, these people now weigh more and have more health issues related to being overweight than people from the area born just three or six months later (Tobi et al., 2014).

## Epigenetics

Scientists struggled to reconcile this and other new evidence with the genetic theory they knew. They hypothesized that while the blueprint for a building is unchanging and must be followed to the tiniest specifications, our DNA "blueprint" is only partially fixed. Some parts of it are unalterable—for example, the sizes of our feet—but many parts are more like suggestions or possibilities than orders. The exciting new field based on these discoveries is called *epigenetics*, the study of how people's environments and experiences affect the function of their genes. Epigenetic changes are long-lasting modifications in gene function that do not actually change the genetic code. They are the link between environmental and genetic factors (Kubota, Miyake, & Hirasawa, 2012).

In contrast to the DNA sequence, which is static, the epigenome, or the many chemical compounds surrounding the genome and directing its activity, is susceptible to modification. It is, in fact, quite responsive to the environment, to our emotions, and to what we eat. The epigenome is like a light switch that turns on or off the expression of specific genes. Through the epigenome, environmental factors profoundly influence the ways in which genes are expressed. Physical activity and exposure to stress can also switch genes on or off. For example, environmental toxins and viral infections can fuel epigenetic processes that may contribute to the increased prevalence of autism. Both major depressive disorder and bipolar disorder are likely the result of interactions between genes and the environment (Kubota, Miyake, & Hirasawa, 2012).

The starvation studies from the Dutch Hunger Winter demonstrated the existence of a process called transgenerational epigenetic inheritance, by which epigenetic changes can affect the genome of children and even grandchildren (Kubota, Miyake, & Hirasawa, 2012). While some epigenetic changes last a lifetime or longer, others can appear and disappear at any time, in response to diet, weight, stress, or exposure to tobacco or chemicals like DDT (Schardt, 2013).

Changes in gene expression affecting the next generation come not only from the mother. A recent study at Duke University explored the expression of a gene related to growth promotion in 79 newborns. They found the gene was more turned on in those born to obese fathers than to children of fathers of normal weight (Schardt, 2013). The chemical reason that genes do not determine health in a uniform way is that they carry chemical attachments that act on DNA to regulate the timing and amount of the gene without changing its basic composition. These chemical attachments, or epigenetic markers, determine whether a gene is expressed or silenced.

DNA methylation and modification of histones by acetylation are the epigenetic mechanisms by which environmental factors influence genetic expression. Lithium is one of the few factors that can actually induce both mechanisms of turning genes off and on. A methyl group consists of one carbon atom bonded to three hydrogen atoms. DNA methylation is a chemical process that attaches a methyl group of atoms directly to a DNA strand, thereby preventing expression of the gene (Simmons, 2008). The Dutch babies in early gestation during the famine experienced less methylation of the growth gene than babies at a later gestational age. Those babies born six months later did not experience the same lack of methylation. When enough methyl groups attach to a gene, they can turn the gene OFF. Methylation does not affect the gene itself but only the degree to which the gene will be translated into protein.

Acetylation is the other important mechanism that affects gene expression. If enough acetyl groups—each of these consists of two carbon atoms, one oxygen atom, and three hydrogen atoms—become attached to a histone, the gene may get switched ON. Histones are complex proteins that function as spools for threads of DNA to wrap around. Changes in the chemical structure of these proteins immediately affect the way genes are expressed (Simmons, 2008).

## Nutrigenomics

Nutrigenomics, a new field of study, is focused on identifying dietary factors that have an effect on the expression of genes. Nutrients are powerful environmental factors because they communicate with genetic material and influence biological responses. Nutrients can modify the expression of genes associated with physiologic and pathologic processes like aging and carcinogenesis. Knowledge of nutrigenomics can lead to the evolving reality of true personalized medicine. For instance, if a patient is susceptible to chronic inflammation, a diet high in omega-3 fats can be helpful to reduce the expression of genes that code for inflammatory cytokines, thereby reducing the inflammatory response. The understanding of nutrigenomics will lead to individualized recommendations for the prevention and treatment of many chronic diseases (Gropper & Smith, 2012).

Nutrients and bioactive food components (e.g., flavonoids, carotenoids) can directly inhibit enzymes that catalyze DNA methylation or histone modifications. Indeed, folate, vitamin B12, methionine, and choline can affect DNA methylation and histone acetylation. Epigenetics has been implicated in a range of diseases including obesity, immune diseases, and now neurocognitive disorders. Folate is a B vitamin that is essential for the maintenance of DNA methylation. Folic acid supplements can alter DNA methylation status and are recommended for pregnant women because folic acid prevents neural tube defects such as spina bifida. Folic acid supplements can have a positive effect on several features of autism in children, although the underlying mechanism is not completely understood. Folic acid likely exerts a global effect on the genome (Kubota, Miyake, & Hirasawa, 2012).

## Epigenetics and Psychiatry

The new field of epigenetics has far-reaching implications for psychiatry. First, it gives a new perspective to the meaning of an inherited disorder. As acquired epigenetic alterations can be transferred to the next generations, what scientists used to label as an inherited psychiatric disease may in fact be the result of epigenetic changes in a family's shared environment. Many psychiatric diseases are consistent with the theory of epigenetic dysregulation because of their fluctuating nature and disease course.

Single gene and whole genome epigenetic analyses have shown atypical epigenetic markers in the blood or brain of individuals with psychiatric diseases, including abnormalities in DNA methylation, histone modifications and microRNA expression. Many psychiatric treatments such as valproate, lithium, and electroconvulsive therapy alter epigenetic codes. Lithium can increase histone acetylation and decrease DNA methylation in responders (Mostafavi, Abdolmaleky, 2014).

Among genes that potentially protect against the development of mood disorders, the brain derived neurotrophic factor (BDNF) gene has been the focus of study for the past several years, as it is associated with neural development and proliferation. BDNF is the most prevalent growth factor in the central nervous system. Because it plays a critical role in the development of plasticity of the brain, methylation of BDNF takes a toll on brain health and resilience. The BDNF gene seems to modulate how much or how little environmental experiences—for instance pharmacological treatment, exercise, or exposure to stress—become encoded within the neurons and neural circuits and thereby lead to long-lasting effects. This protein promotes the growth and formation of new neurons, and it may be responsible in part for the remarkable effect of exercise on the brain and for the increase in hippocampus size that is linked with improved memory (D'Addario et al., 2012).

Conversely, mood disorders are often associated with methylation of BDNF. Adverse experiences like major depression can lower BDNF levels and are linked with hippocampal shrinkage, a phenomenon that helps explain some of the cognitive impairments that are a hallmark of depression. Studies have revealed higher levels of DNA methylation at the BDNF gene promoter in patients with major depressive disorder and bipolar disorder II compared to levels in patients with bipolar I (Dell'Osso et al., 2014).

Extreme methylation is also apparent in the DNA of patients with other psychiatric issues. Evidence of methylation has been observed in patients who suffered childhood adversity (Labonte et al., 2012). The effects of broad reprogramming caused by severe DNA methylation have been found in the hippocampi of suicide victims. In fact, in one study, hippocampal DNA from the brains of people who had completed suicide revealed DNA methylation changes at more than 300 gene loci. Striking differences in DNA methylation between suicide completers and comparison subjects in this study strongly suggest that DNA methylation fuels particular behavior changes leading to suicide (Labonte et al., 2013).

But if the effects of methylation on the DNA of people with psychiatric disorders look bleak, the promise lies in the fact that epigenetic changes are reversible. While the larger field of genetics has often seemed deterministic, new insights from epigenetics are instead empowering. In some areas psychiatric treatment is already focusing on the epigenome and changes in gene expression. Epigenetic programming caused by early unfortunate experiences has been shown to be reversible by positive psychosocial experiences. The great promise of epigenetics is that if harmful changes in gene expression are reversible, epigenetics can also be used to restore health. Scientists are now exploring how to dim the expression of genes that lead to disease or mental disorders while stimulating the expression of health-enhancing genes through nutritional and pharmaceutical intervention.

## Lithium's Influences on Genes

Lithium deficiency is one of the most common mineral deficiencies associated with nearly every type of psychiatric disorder. Lithium is a powerful epigenetic factor that can be used to subdue the expression of genes that lead to disease or mental disorders while fostering the expression of health-enhancing genes.

Lithium exerts extensive genetic changes that are unique and not fully understood, as there are likely many more genetic changes we are not aware of. Genes that are significantly altered by lithium treatment are involved many functions such as cell communication, immune response, protein metabolism, nucleic acid regulation/metabolism, and cell growth and maintenance. A study of rat frontal cortex showed chronic treatment with lithium led to the significant up-regulation of 57 genes and down-regulation of 151 genes. Four of those genes have been specifically associated with bipolar disorder (Fatemi, Reutiman, & Folsom, 2009).

Lithium changes gene expression through two basic channels: DNA methylation, and acetylation or histone modification. Lithium acts by preventing the process of DNA methylation, which is critically important to improving mental health and preventing mental and emotional disorders. At least three studies have demonstrated that lithium decreases DNA methylation of the BDNF gene promoter. In other words, lithium increases the expression of the BDNF gene.

The increased synthesis of BDNF contributes to robust neural growth and healthy dendritic branching. In one study of hippocampal neurons, lithium increased mRNA expression of BDNF by 67%. At a higher lithium dose there was a 100% increase. Likewise, the protein level of BDNF was increased by 53% with the lower lithium dose and by 89% with the higher lithium dose. By ensuring that the BDNF gene is left in the "on" position, lithium promotes the consistent release of protective neurotrophins that protect and nourish the brain (Dwivedi & Zhang, 2015).

BDNF levels are diminished both in the brain and serum of Alzheimer's patients. Alzheimer's patients treated for ten weeks with lithium showed a significant increase in their BDNF serum levels. They also saw a significant decrease of cognitive impairment compared with placebo-treated Alzheimer's patients. Reduction of cognitive impairment was inversely correlated with lithium serum concentration (Leyhe et al., 2009).

BDNF contributes to degradation of amyloid-β, a component of the amyloid plaques found in the brains of Alzheimer's patients. In addition, BDNF is capable of inactivating GSK3β (Leyhe et al., 2009). Abnormal regulation and expression of GSK3β is associated with an increased susceptibility to Alzheimer's disease and bipolar disorder. Lithium's ability to enhance the synthesis of BDNF has exciting implications for improving a wide range of neuropsychiatric disorders.

Lithium also acts through histone modification. Histone function is particularly important for the encoding of high-level cognitive functions like learning and memory. In fact, diminished memory, as seen in patients with Alzheimer's disease, has been linked to problems with histone metabolism. In experiments with laboratory animals, lithium has been shown to increase histone acetylation by weakening the binding of the DNA to its spool, making it more available to proteins that enhance memory (Lee et al., 2015). Although studies in humans are needed to further delineate the exact mechanism, lithium may be beneficial in preventing the genetic changes associated with the development of Alzheimer's disease and other neurodegenerative conditions.

These biological mechanisms are also important in lithium's role in the treatment of bipolar disorder. Lithium affects multiple pathways in the brain, which may explain its efficacy and the underlying pathophysiology of bipolar disorder. BDNF has been consistently reported to be decreased in bipolar patients. One study found that bipolar patients had significantly lower BDNF levels during mania and depression compared to euthymic patients and healthy controls. However, for those on lithium treatment, BDNF levels correlated positively with lithium levels (Tunca, 2014).

Important findings come from a study that looked into lithium-induced alterations in genome-wide gene expression profiles within the mRNA of fruit flies. The fly model is relevant because the genetic pathways involved in lithium's actions in the nervous system appear to be shared by fruit flies and higher vertebrates. Two genes were downregulated and 14 were upregulated in response to lithium treatment. The expression of genes that are related to amino acid metabolism is significantly affected by lithium treatment. The degradation pathways for branched-chain amino acids (BCAAs) are specifically enhanced by lithium treatment. One possible implication of this is a change in brain serotonin level. Serotonin is synthesized from tryptophan in neurons so brain tryptophan levels play a critical role in the availability of serotonin. All large neutral amino acids, such as tryptophan and BCAAs, are transported into the brain across the blood-brain barrier by a single transport system. All of these amino acids compete for the carrier proteins. This means that lower levels of BCAAs result in higher tryptophan (and consequently higher serotonin) levels in the brain. Reduced brain serotonin activity is thought to contribute to the pathogenesis of mood disorders. The tryptophan-to-BCAA ratio is significantly lower in unipolar and bipolar patients than in control subjects. It is likely that modulation of amino acids contributes to lithium's therapeutic action (Kasuya, Kaas, & Kitamoto, 2009).

The field of epigenetics is in its infancy, but we already know that lithium promotes epigenetic modifications that affect the expression of more than 50 genes, including signaling proteins, transcription factors, activators, cell adhesion proteins, oncogenes, and tumor suppressors (Farah et al., 2013). As research expands our knowledge of how to manipulate gene expression and suppression, targeted use of lithium will enable us to prevent and treat psychiatric disorders that now incapacitate those who suffer from them. By acting directly on the epigenome, lithium restores neural function and improves brain health in ways that just a few years ago were not dreamed possible.

## CHAPTER 6 | References

D'Addario, C., Dell'Osso, B., Palazzo, M. C., Benatti, B., Lietti, L., Cattaneo, E., & ... Altamura, A. C. (2012). Selective DNA methylation of BDNF promoter in bipolar disorder: Differences among patients with BDI and BDII. *Neuropsychopharmacology, 37*(7), 1647-1655.

Dell'Osso, B., D'Addario, C., Carlotta Palazzo, M., Benatti, B., Camuri, G., Galimberti, D., & ... Carlo Altamura, A. (2014). Epigenetic modulation of BDNF gene: differences in DNA methylation between unipolar and bipolar patients. *Journal of Affective Disorders, 166*, 330-333.

Dwivedi, T., & Zhang, H. (2015). Lithium-induced neuroprotection is associated with epigenetic modification of specific BDNF gene promoter and altered expression of apoptotic-regulatory proteins. *Frontiers in Neuroscience, 8*, 457.

Farah, R., Khamisy-Farah, R., Amit, T., Youdim, M. H., & Arraf, Z. (2013). Lithium's Gene Expression Profile, Relevance to Neuroprotection A cDNA Microarray Study. *Cellular and Molecular Neurobiology, 33*(3), 411.

Fatemi, S. H., Reutiman, T. J., & Folsom, T. D. (2009). The role of lithium in modulation of brain genes: relevance for aetiology and treatment of bipolar disorder. *Biochemical Society Transactions, 37*(Pt 5), 1090-1095.

Gropper, S. S., & Smith, J. S. (2012). *Advanced Nutrition and Human Metabolism*. 6th ed. Belmont, CA: Wadsworth Publishing.

Kasuya, J., Kaas, G., & Kitamoto, T. (2009). Effects of lithium chloride on the gene expression profiles in Drosophila heads. *Neuroscience Research, 6*(4), 413-420.

Kubota, T., Miyake, K., & Hirasawa, T. (2012). Epigenetic understanding of gene-environment interactions in psychiatric disorders: a new concept of clinical genetics. *Clinical Epigenetics, 4*(1), 1.

Labonte, B., Suderman, M., Maussion, G., Navaro, L., Yerko, V., Mahar, I., & ... Turecki, G. (2012). Genome-wide epigenetic regulation by early-life trauma. *Archives of General Psychiatry, 69*(7), 722-731.

Labonte, B., Suderman, M., Maussion, G., Lopez, J. P., Navarro-Sánchez, L., Yerko, V., & . Turecki, G. (2013). Genome-wide methylation changes in the brains of suicide completers. *American Journal of Psychiatry, 170*(5), 511-520.

Lee, R. S., Pirooznia, M., Guintivano, J., Ly, M., Ewald, E. R., Tamashiro, K. L., & ... Potash, J. B. (2015). Search for common targets of lithium and valproic acid identifies novel epigenetic effects of lithium on the rat leptin receptor gene. *Translational Psychiatry, 5*, e600.

Leyhe, T., Eschweiler, G. W., Stransky, E., Gasser, T., Annas, P., Basun, H., & Laske, C. (2009). Increase of BDNF serum concentration in lithium treated patients with early Alzheimer's disease. *Journal of Alzheimer's Disease, 16*(3), 649-656.

Mostafavi Abdolmaleky, H. (2014). Horizons of psychiatric genetics and epigenetics: where are we and where are we heading? *Iranian Journal of Psychiatry and Behavioral Sciences, 8*(3), 1-10.

Simmons, D. (2008). Epigenetic influences and disease. *Nature Education, 1*(1), 6.

Schardt, D. (2013). Epigenetics: It's what turns you on..and off. *Nutrition Action Health Letter, 40*(6), 9-11.

Tobi, E. W., Goeman, J. J., Monajemi, R., Gu, H., Putter, H., Zhang, Y., & ... Heijmans, B. T. (2014). DNA methylation signatures link prenatal famine exposure to growth and metabolism. *Nature Communications, 5*, 5592.

Tunca, Z., Ozerdem, A., Ceylan, D., Yalçın, Y., Can, G., Resmi, H., & ... Kerim, D. (2014). Alterations in BDNF (brain derived neurotrophic factor) and GDNF (glial cell line-derived neurotrophic factor) serum levels in bipolar disorder: The role of lithium. *Journal of Affective Disorders, 166*, 193-200.

# Seven

## LITHIUM AS A MEDICINE: DEMENTIA & ALZHEIMER'S DISEASE

The human brain, with its impressive capacity to create, imagine and solve complex problems, also seems to have a surprising physiological tendency towards deterioration. Our longer life span and larger brain size seem to come with an evolutionary price: as far as researchers can tell, humans are the only animals vulnerable to neurodegenerative brain disorders such as Alzheimer's disease.

Every 67 seconds someone in the United States develops Alzheimer's disease. This year 700,000 individuals over the age of 65 will die with dementia. Last year friends and family of people with Alzheimer's and other dementias provided an estimated 17.9 billion hours of unpaid care to their family members or friends with the disease (WHO, 2015; Alzheimer's Association, 2015).

Neurodegenerative disorders have become an international public health issue with devastating medical, social, and economic consequences. And yet, from the perspective of conventional medicine, almost nothing is known about how to treat or stop them. In the midst of a harrowing race to find answers, one unassuming prevention strategy has shown promise above the rest. This remedy is none other than the simple, brain-protecting nutrient: lithium.

## Understanding Dementia and Alzheimer's

Alzheimer's disease is a tragic neurological malady characterized by a progressive and irreparable shrinking of brain tissue. The result is a devastating decline in memory, social abilities, and communication skills in sufferers resulting, eventually, in death. Worldwide an estimated 35.6 million people currently live with Alzheimer's disease or a similar neurodegenerative disorder, and these numbers are on a staggering rise. The World Health Organization has projected that this troublesome statistic will double by 2030 (65.7 million) and triple by the year 2050 (115.4 million). Already in America, Alzheimer's disease is the sixth leading cause of death; one in three seniors perishes with this type of crippling memory loss (WHO, 2015).

The human brain has billions of brain cells or neurons that work in collaboration to manage varying aspects of cognitive function. Distinct networks of neurons, or regions of the brain, are responsible for specific processes like memory, emotion, or movement. When the cells become compromised or injured in any one area, that region is left unable to carry out its designated roles effectively. Our modern world is filled with dangers that threaten our neurons. Toxin exposure, traumatic brain injury, lack of blood flow, or oxidative stress can all cause damage to brain cells. When neurons are compromised in some way, and certain areas of the brain no longer function optimally, the condition is called dementia. In other words, dementia is not a specific disease—but rather a broad term used to describe the range of neurodegenerative symptoms that manifest with a loss of brain cell function.

Core mental skills that are impaired in dementia may include:

- Short term memory
- Judgment and problem solving
- Communication and language
- Ability to focus and pay attention
- Visuospatial perception

Traits of dementia vary significantly depending on the location and type of neuronal injury. The hippocampus, a small structure located near the center of the brain, is an area with a particularly high vulnerability to cellular damage. This region is primarily associated with memory and spatial navigation, and is the first location harmed with Alzheimer's disease. Alzheimer's disease is a progressive form of cognitive decline that accounts for approximately 60-80% of all dementia cases (Alzheimer's Association, 2015). In preliminary phases of the disease, memory loss is generally mild, whereas in later stages individuals become increasingly disoriented. Alzheimer's culminates in volatile mood and behavior shifts, and an eventual loss of ability to communicate and interact appropriately within the environment. Finally, the disease ends in death

## Plaques and Tangles in the Brain

In the body, Alzheimer's disease is characterized by a massive and progressive loss of brain tissue. At the cellular level, these changes are the result of two trademark injuries or lesions: plaques and tangles.

Plaques are formed by deposits of small protein fragments called amyloid-$\beta$ or beta-amyloid peptides. Clumps of these proteins form blockages in the spaces between neurons, called the synapses. With the synapses barricaded, normal cell-to-cell signaling cannot occur, and communication is essentially stopped in certain regions of the brain. The physiological processes required for memory and learning are halted, and symptoms begin to arise. Furthermore, the accumulation of beta-amyloid peptides at cell junctions activates the immune system and triggers the inflammatory response. This amplifies interneuronal congestion and spreads damages to disrupt surrounding cells in other areas of the brain. Eventually entire networks of neurons die off and dissolve.

While plaques form in the synapses between cells, other lesions, called neurofibrillary tangles, develop within the neurons themselves. These tangles result from a disruption in the production of a different type of protein, called tau. Normally, tau protein filaments are responsible for reinforcing the microtubules that circulate nutrients and other essential supplies throughout the cell. When tau proteins (also called P-tau) are functioning optimally, they act similarly to the ties on railroad tracks— providing a structure that keeps trains running smoothly and the delivery of their goods on schedule. In Alzheimer's disease, however, the phosphorylation of tau proteins becomes hyperactive and the strands destabilize, becoming twisted or "tangled". The tracks malfunction and eventually start to deteriorate. Without this system to circulate vital compounds, neurons "starve" or die.

The atrophy of brain tissue observed in Alzheimer's disease is thus the result of three overlapping abnormal processes:

- Amyloid plaques form between neurons, creating congestion and blocking communication.
- Tau proteins within nerve cells mutate and disrupt normal intracellular activity.
- Inflammatory cascades are triggered, damaging surrounding tissues.

## What Causes Alzheimer's Disease?

Less than five percent of the time, Alzheimer's disease results from a specific genetic vulnerability that increases the likelihood a person will develop the disease. More commonly, plaques and tangles result from a complex combination of subtle genetic, lifestyle and environmental factors that affect the brain over a lifetime. Scientists believe that Alzheimer's disease is not an acute condition, but rather the result of numerous damages that occur over the years. This slow, cumulative patterning helps to explain why most patients with Alzheimer's disease don't present with symptoms until over the age of 65.

There is now evidence to show that beta-amyloid plaques may actually be a relatively common malformation in the aging human brain. New research is revealing that plaques can appear 30 to 40 years before symptoms of cognitive decline begin to appear (Langbaum, 2013). One recent study published in the *Journal of the American Medical Association* reported that ten percent of healthy 50-year-olds have amyloid deposits. The percentage of amyloid deposits increases to 33% at the age of 80, and 44% at the age of 90 (Visser et al., 2015).

The destruction of the human brain can occur over many years, even when memory and cognitive processes are still intact. Given this level of scientific understanding, it would seem that devising a treatment strategy for Alzheimer's disease should be relatively straightforward: find a way to prevent the formation of plaques and tangles. Unfortunately, the search for a cure has not been so simple.

## The Search for a Cure

A swarm of clinical trials have been launched in recent years, all with the goal of finding effective pharmacological interventions to stop or slow the progression of neurodegenerative disorders like Alzheimer's disease. However between the years 2002 and 2012, 99.6% of drugs studies aimed at preventing, curing, or improving Alzheimer's symptoms were either halted or discontinued (Devlin, 2015). Most of the tested drugs were making patients sicker, not better, and came with disabling side effects.

A recent shift has occurred in the harrowing race to find a cure. The new evidence that plaques begin to accumulate in the brain years *before* symptoms of cognitive decline start has helped scientists realize that although efforts have been well-intentioned, it makes little sense to expend all available resources trying to create a medication that will treat an illness which started decades beforehand. By the time a diagnosis is established with current screening techniques, the internal damage is substantial, if not largely irreversible by pharmaceuticals.

Researchers and clinicians have recognized that what is needed instead is a therapy to strengthen and protect the brain from damage; something with the capacity to prevent the formation of plaques and tangles before the destruction impairs memory and behavior. The optimal solution would be safe and effective, and would offer neuroprotective and neurogenerative properties.

Biotechnological companies have raised billions of dollars in futile attempts to find a preventative neuroprotective treatment. With so many individuals and communities suffering, the stakes are high and so are the investments. Yet while the precious dollars from governments, charity organizations, and generous donors are being gambled away on these trials, scientific literature has already clearly identified that the mineral lithium can do all of this, and more. The only problem is that it isn't patentable, and therefore it isn't profitable. Although the financial incentive for research is minimal, the potential for relief from deteriorating brain health is enormous.

## Lithium: The Unlikely Answer

Lithium salts have been used for centuries as a popular health tonic. Over the course of history this simple mineral has been applied to heal ailments as wide-ranging as asthma, gout, and migraines. In modern medicine, lithium is most widely acknowledged for its ability to encourage mood stability in patients with affective disorders. With years of research and clinical use to back it, a substantial body of evidence now exists to show that lithium restores brain and nervous system function.

So what would happen if this mineral was used with dementia? Could it prevent the development of detrimental plaques and tangles? Could it reverse cognitive losses? And if so, could it do so safely, without side effects?

Studies expounding the neuroprotective potential of lithium have been present in the scientific literature for decades, but it wasn't until recently that a small group of researchers began to take notice of a clinical trend specifically linking lithium to the prevention of cognitive decline. Interest was first piqued by providers, who were repeatedly reporting that their bipolar patients taking lithium to stabilize mood also seemed to have decreased rates of Alzheimer's disease later in life.

In an attempt to better understand this link, one study compared the rates of Alzheimer's disease in 66 elderly patients with bipolar disorder and chronic lithium therapy, with the occurrence in 48 similar patients who were not prescribed the mineral. Findings in favor of lithium were staggering: patients receiving continuous lithium showed a decreased prevalence of Alzheimer's disease (5%) as compared with those in the non-lithium group (33%) (Nunes et al., 2007). Two further studies in Denmark confirmed this phenomenon using different study designs, but achieving strikingly similar results. In this study series, investigators surveyed the records of over 21,000 patients who had received lithium treatment, and found that the therapy was associated with decreased levels of both dementia and Alzheimer's (Kessing et al., 2008; Kessing et al., 2010).

# Lithium as a Medicine: Dementia & Alzheimer's Disease

Unfortunately, the first clinical trials testing lithium with dementia patients proved disappointing. Researchers attempted to fit lithium into the same diagnostic treatment framework used by drug companies in the beginning: testing the therapy on patients who already had fully developed Alzheimer's. At this point, the damages to the brain were simply too great to turn around.

One small, open-label study looked at low dose lithium use in 22 Alzheimer's disease patients over the course of one year (MacDonald et al., 2008). These patients had advanced cognitive decline secondary to Alzheimer's disease. While researchers concluded that prescription lithium salts were relatively safe in this population, there were no observed cognitive benefits. The baseline sample size was small and there was a high discontinuation rate. It is clear that the intervention was too late for lithium to make a difference in the advanced stages of illness where plaques and neurofibrillary tangles are already embedded in the neuronal architecture.

Another multi-center, single-blind study looked at the use of lithium sulfate in participants with mild Alzheimer's disease only over a 10 week period (Hampel, 2009). They too failed to find significant effects of lithium treatment on cognitive performance or related biomarkers. The major issue with this trial, however, was the length of observation. It will take months, not weeks, to see substantial cognitive shifts in patients who have developed a disease over 30 years.

A group led by Forlenza et al (2011) sought to correct for these initial design flaws. Focus was shifted away from the post-diagnosis period and settled on prevention. This unique study attempted to determine whether long-term lithium treatment could stop Alzheimer's disease from occurring in high-risk individuals. Forty-five participants with mild cognitive impairment (MCI), a precursor to Alzheimer's, were randomized to receive lithium or a placebo. Over the 12-month trial, lithium dosages were kept at sub-therapeutic levels (150mg to 600mg daily) to minimize potential side effects. At the conclusion of the study, researchers discovered that those in the lithium group had a decreased presence of destructive tau proteins when compared to pre-study levels. This finding came in stark contrast to the tau levels of the placebo group, which had increased steadily over the course of the study. What's more, the lithium group showed improved performance on multiple cognitive scales.

Overall tolerability of lithium was deemed good as patients reported limited side effects, and the adherence rate to treatment was an impressive 91%. Researchers concluded that lithium had a significant disease-modifying impact on preventing dementia and Alzheimer's disease when initiated early in the disease progression.

Additional research has found that lithium may be even most effective when used at micro-doses or supplemental levels, similar to those found naturally in water and foods. In a study published in *Alzheimer's Research*, a scant 0.3 mg of lithium was administered once daily to Alzheimer's patients for 15 months (Nunes, 2013). Those receiving lithium demonstrated stable cognitive performance scores throughout the duration of the study, while those in the control group suffered progressive declines. Moreover, 3 months into the study, the seemingly impossible happened: the symptoms of Alzheimer's disease in these patients actually improved! The lithium treatment cohort began showing increasing scores on a standardized test assessing cognitive function.

These findings further support the incredible potential of lithium, not only for stopping the on-going deterioration seen in dementia, but even for encouraging cognitive repair when used early in treatment.

## How Lithium Works In the Brain

Indeed many of lithium's benefits for use in Alzheimer's are the result of its general neuroprotective and neurogenerative effects, which are outlined in detail in Chapters 5 and 6. Below is a review of Alzheimer's- specific mechanisms that lithium targets and protects.

### *Lithium Inhibits Glycogen-Synthase Kinase-3 (GSK3)*

Lithium modifies activity of the enzyme Glycogen Synthase Kinase-3 (GSK3). In the nervous system, GSK3 helps to coordinate neural growth and development by activating proteins in the cells. This versatile enzyme is also important for synaptic remodeling, the biological process that drives memory formation. This makes GSK3 of particular importance when it comes to understanding Alzheimer's disease. (Jope & Roh, 2006;Hooper et al., 2008).

# Lithium as a Medicine: Dementia & Alzheimer's Disease

Researchers have found that in Alzheimer's patients, GSK3 activity is excessively high in the areas of the brain that control memory and behavior, such as the hippocampus and frontal cortex. Experts predict that GSK3 phosphorylates, or activates, proteins in these regions at too rapid a rate. Amyloid-β and tau proteins are among the key proteins activated. They begin to accumulate, creating signature plaques, and neurofibrillary tangles form in the brain tissue.

Finding ways to inhibit GSK3 has been an area of focus for Alzheimer's researchers. Luckily, lithium is a well-established GSK3 inhibitor. By dimming GSK3 activity, lithium may slow the production of amyloid and tau proteins, and prevent related damages. (Hooper et al., 2008; Wada, 2009; Engel et al., 2006).

### *LITHIUM REMOVES PLAQUES AND TANGLES FROM CELLS*

In addition to slowing amyloid-β and tau protein production, lithium promotes their removal from cells by repairing damaged "cleaning systems" in the neurons. Nerve cells regularly undergo the process of autophagy, wherein unwanted or dysfunctional cell components are broken down and removed. However, in Alzheimer's and other neurodegenerative diseases, autophagy is disabled. When autophagy is blocked, amyloid peptides and tau protein can accumulate much faster and with more destructive effects (Cheung, 2011).

Lithium salts have been shown to stimulate autophagy. Lithium therefore corrects the waste removal process in cells so that lesion-causing proteins are eliminated (Sarkar, et al., 2005; Ravikumar, et al., 2010).

### *LITHIUM PREVENTS NEURONAL DESTRUCTION*

When cells are too damaged to be cleaned or repaired, a cell death program is normally activated. The targeted cell shrinks, condenses, and disassembles in a neat way so that no harm is caused to neighboring cells. In Alzheimer's disease apoptosis can be helpful in for clearing cells that have become overrun with misfolded proteins and can no longer carry out their duties.

The problem is that apoptosis becomes dysregulated in many Alzheimer's patients. Cell death is triggered in random nervous system cells (Shimohama, 2000). Lithium acts to counterbalance this effect by suppressing the pro-apoptotic molecules that initiate the cell death program. Simultaneously, lithium ions support the expression of anti-apoptotic molecules, which mark cells as healthy so that they are not mistaken as candidates for apoptosis. (Manji, 1999; Chen et al., 1999; Liechti et al., 2014).

By recalibrating the rate of apoptosis, or cell death, in the nervous system, lithium can slow the accelerated tissue loss that accompanies Alzheimer's disease and other neurodegenerative illnesses.

### *LITHIUM REGULATES GLUTAMATE*

Glutamate is generally considered the most important neurotransmitter for normal brain function. It is estimated that over half of all brain synapses release the chemical glutamate as a means to communicate. However, because glutamate is a strong excitatory chemical, it is important that it is swiftly cleared from the nerve cell junctions to keep messages brief. An excess of glutamate can overwhelm the neurons, leading to agitation, injury, and eventually cell death (Hamilton et al., 2015). This often occurs in Alzheimer's disease, wherein an overabundance of excitatory glutamate floods the cells.

Lithium prevents the uptake of glutamate into the cells by deactivating N-methyl-D-aspartate (NMDA) receptors, the main class of glutamate receptors in the nervous tissue. This action protects the neurons from its potential excitotoxic effects (Hashimoto et al., 2002).

Balancing intracellular glutamate levels is another pathway through which lithium may prevent cell death associated with Alzheimer's disease and related symptoms of cognitive decline.

## Low Dose Lithium Therapy

The pharmaceutical industry remains committed to developing expensive, patentable drugs for dementia. Indeed, such treatments, if given to large numbers of people over long periods of time, would be quite lucrative. However to date, none of them have proven to be successful.

Low dose lithium on the other hand appears to be a preventative agent, and yet with no patent and a limited ability to sell, it has not gained the attention it deserves. Although a few solid clinical trials have been completed, the research potential has been limited and severely undercut by a lack of vested funding. Commercial interest has remained pitifully low, and as a result, few clinicians have been exposed to the research on how to use low dose lithium in practice.

However, if we look behind the politics and put together the evidence we do have, lithium's role in preventing cognitive decline becomes even clearer. Data exists to show that the mineral lithium is important for neuroprotection, repair of cells, and neurogenesis throughout the life span. Lithium deficiency is known to be deleterious to neuronal health, and its administration at nutritional doses results in clinically relevant improvements in neurological conditions.

## Understanding Lithium's Role in Preventing Cognitive Decline

Alzheimer's and dementia have become modern health problems of epidemic proportions. Nonetheless, relatively few pharmacological solutions have been discovered for preventing, treating, and reversing associated cognitive decline.

Emerging evidence suggests that simple low dose lithium may play a key role in shifting the pathophysiological cascade associated with dementia and Alzheimer's disease. In clinical studies, long-term lithium therapy has been found to decrease the problematic plaques and tangles leading to symptoms of cognitive decline. This powerful mineral acts by inhibiting damaging enzymes, increasing autophagic processes in neurons, and stimulating the release of protective neurotrophic factors in the brain. Lithium ions have been found to operate most efficiently at low doses mimicking those found in nutritional sources. At these sub-pharmaceutical levels, lithium has been shown to be a beneficial and safe neuroprotective therapy across age groups and with minimal side effects.

The safety profile of low dose lithium is particularly attractive, as prevention strategies for dementia are most effective when started early and continued for long periods of time. The dangerous plaques and tangles involved in Alzheimer's disease start up to 40 years before the appearance of symptoms. What's more, 10% of healthy 50 year olds already have amyloid deposits in the brain tissues. Thus for optimal effectiveness, steps to protect the brain must be taken at a much younger age than previously thought.

When started early, low dose lithium may be the key intervention to prevent cognitive decline.

## CHAPTER 7 | References

Alzheimer's Association. (2015). Alzheimer's disease facts and figures. *Alzheimer's & Dementia: The Journal of the Alzheimer's Association, 11*(3), 332.

Chen, D. F., Schneider, G. E., Martinou, J., & Tonegawa, S. (1997). Bcl-2 promotes regeneration of severed axons in mammalian CNS. *Nature, 385*(6615), 434-439.

Chen, G., Zeng, W. Z., Yuan, P. X., Huang, L. D., Jiang, Y. M., Zhao, Z. H., & Manji, H. K. (1999). The mood-stabilizing agents lithium and valproate robustly increase the levels of the neuroprotective protein bcl-2 in the CNS. *Journal of Neurochemistry, 72*(2), 879-882.

Cheung, Z. H., & Ip, N. Y. (2011). Autophagy deregulation in neurodegenerative diseases - recent advances and future perspectives. *Journal of Neurochemistry, 118*(3), 317.

Devlin, H. (2015, July 22). Scientists find first drug that appears to slow Alzheimer's disease. *The Guardian.* Retrieved from www.theguardian.com/science/2015/jul/22/scientists-find-first-drug-slow-alzheimers-disease

Engel, T., Goni-Oliver, P., Lucas, J. J., Avila, J., & Hernandez, F. (2006). Chronic lithium administration to FTDP-17 tau and GSK-3beta overexpressing mice prevents tau hyperphosphorylation and neurofibrillary tangle formation, but pre-formed neurofibrillary tangles do not revert. *Journal of Neurochemistry, 99*(6), 1445-55.

Forlenza, O. V., Diniz, B. S., Radanovic, M., Santos, F. S., Talib, L. L., & Gattaz, W. F. (2011). Disease modifying properties of long-term lithium treatment for amnestic mild cognitive impairment: Randomised controlled trial. *British Journal of Psychiatry, 198*(5), 351-356.

Hamilton, A., Zamponi, G. W., & Ferguson, S. G. (2015). Glutamate receptors function as scaffolds for the regulation of β-amyloid and cellular prion protein signaling complexes. *Molecular Brain, 8,* 18.

Hampel, H., Ewers, M., Bürger, K., Annas, P., Mörtberg, A., Bogstedt, A., & ... Basun, H. (2009). Lithium trial in Alzheimer's disease: A randomized, single-blind, placebo-controlled, multicenter 10-week study. *Journal of Clinical Psychiatry, 70*(6), 922-931.

Harwood, A. J. (2005). Lithium and bipolar mood disorder: The inositol-depletion hypothesis revisited. *Molecular Psychiatry, 10*(1), 117-126.

Hashimoto, R., Hough, C., Nakazawa, T., Yamamoto, T., & Chuang, D. (2002). Lithium protection against glutamate excitotoxicity in rat cerebral cortical neurons: involvement of NMDA receptor inhibition possibly by decreasing NR2B tyrosine phosphorylation. *Journal of Neurochemistry, 80*(4), 589-597.

Hooper, C., Killick, R., & Lovestone, S. (2008). The GSK3 hypothesis of Alzheimer's disease. *Journal of Neurochemistry, 104*(6), 1433.

Jansen, W. J., Ossenkoppele, R., Knol, D. L., Tijms, B. M., Scheltens, P., Verhey, F. R., & Visser, P. J. (2015). Prevalence of cerebral amyloid pathology in persons without dementia: a meta-analysis. *JAMA, 313*(19), 1924-1938.

Jope, R. S., & Roh, M. (2006). Glycogen synthase kinase-3 (GSK3) in psychiatric diseases and therapeutic interventions. *Current Drug Targets, 7*(11), 1421-1434.

Kessing, L. V., Sondergard, L., Forman, J. L., & Andersen, P. K. (2008). Lithium treatment and risk of dementia. *Archives of General Psychiatry, 65*(11), 1331.

Kessing, L. V., Forman, J. L., & Andersen, P. K. (2010). Does lithium protect against dementia? *Bipolar Disorders, 12*(1), 87.

Langbaum, J. B., Fleisher, A. S., Chen, K., Ayutyanont, N., Lopera, F., Quiroz, Y. T., & ... Reiman, E. M. (2013). Ushering in the study and treatment of preclinical Alzheimer disease. *Nature Reviews Neurology, 9*(7), 371.

Liechti, F. D., Südle, N., Theurillat, R., Grandgirard, D., Thormann, W., & Leib, S. L. (2014). The mood-stabilizer lithium prevents hippocampal apoptosis and improves spatial memory in experimental meningitis. *Plos One, 9*(11), e113607.

Macdonald, A., Briggs, K., Poppe, M., Higgins, A., Velayudhan, L., & Lovestone, S. (2008). A feasibility and tolerability study of lithium in

Alzheimer's disease. *International Journal of Geriatric Psychiatry, 23*(7), 704-711.

Manji, H. K., Moore, G. J., & Chen, G. (1999). Lithium at 50: Have the neuroprotective effects of this unique cation been overlooked? *Biological Psychiatry, 46*(7), 929-940.

Nunes, M. A., Viel, T. A., & Buck, H. S. (2013). Microdose lithium treatment stabilized cognitive impairment in patients with Alzheimer's disease. *Current Alzheimer Research, 10*(1), 104-107.

Nunes, P. V., Forlenza, O. V., & Gattaz, W. F. (2007). Lithium and risk for Alzheimer's disease in elderly patients with bipolar disorder. *British Journal of Psychiatry, 190*, 359-360.

Sarkar, S., Floto, R. A., Berger, Z., Imarisio, S., Cordenier, A., Pasco, M., & Rubinsztein, D. C. (2005). Lithium Induces Autophagy by Inhibiting Inositol Monophosphatase. *Journal of Cell Biology, 170*(7), 1101-11.

Shimohama, S. (2000). Apoptosis in Alzheimer's disease—an update. *Apoptosis, 5*(1), 9-16.

Ravikumar, B., Sarkar, S., Davies, J. E., Futter, M., Garcia-Arencibia, M., Green-Thompson, Z. W., & ... Rubinsztein, D. C. (2010). Regulation of mammalian autophagy in physiology and pathophysiology. *Physiological Reviews, 90*(4), 1383-435.

Wada, A. (2009). Lithium and neuropsychiatric therapeutics: neuroplasticity via glycogen synthase kinase-3beta, beta-catenin, and neurotrophin cascades. *Journal of Pharmacological Sciences, 110*(1), 14-28.

World Health Organization (WHO). (2015). *Facts and Figures: Dementia.* Retrieved from: www.who.int/mediacentre/factsheets/fs362/en

# Eight

## LITHIUM AS A MEDICINE: PARKINSON'S DISEASE

Parkinson's disease affects nearly one million individuals in the United States and is the second most common neurodegenerative disorder after Alzheimer's disease (Kowal, 2013). It is a chronic and progressive neurological disorder, characterized by an inability to control movement normally. Currently there is no cure for Parkinson's, although in recent years, a sizeable amount of funding and research have gone into the development of new pharmaceuticals for the disease.

In spite of aggressive treatments, however, progress in therapy for Parkinson's has been slow. This is not surprising, as it takes an average of $1 billion dollars of funding and 15 to 30 years to bring just one central nervous system drug to the market. Scientists are finally starting to explore the curative potential of existing natural substances that would be more readily available to patients in need. The neuroprotective potential of the mineral lithium has been a promising area of research.

We now know that lithium has several important neuroprotective mechanisms that could provide tremendous benefits for Parkinson's patients. For example, lithium ions de-activate the brain damaging enzyme GSK3 that has been implicated in Parkinson's disease pathology. Lithium has also been shown to decrease oxidative stress, bolster antioxidant levels, and increase concentrations of the nervous system preserving protein BDNF. Together, these neuroprotective mechanisms may offset the nerve degeneration that drives the debilitating symptoms of Parkinson's.

Researchers are looking at the potential of using lithium to delay the onset and slow the progression of motor impairments in Parkinson's. Low dose lithium has been especially intriguing, as side effects diminish when the dose decreases. Initial animal studies testing the benefits of low dose lithium on Parkinson's pathology have been promising, and plans for clinical trials in humans are in early stages. Perhaps most intriguing, however, is the evidence that suggests that lithium deficiency may be a contributing factor to the development of Parkinson's in the first place. There is data to show that lithium deficiency is deleterious to neuronal health, and that the administration of lithium results in clinical improvement in individuals with neurological conditions.

As Parkinson's researcher Laurie K. Mischley, ND, MPG, PhD suggests, the most pragmatic question to answer is "If lithium deficiency were not present, would there be fewer cases, less activity or reduced progression of CNS disease?" (Mischley, 2012).

## Understanding Parkinson's Disease

Like Alzheimer's disease, Parkinson's and other neurodegenerative disorders share common pathophysiological processes. The central abnormality in Alzheimer's is an accumulation of abnormal beta-amyloid and tau proteins in the brain tissue. In Parkinson's disease, clumps of a different type of protein, called alpha-synuclein, appear. Anomalous deposits of the alpha-synuclein proteins are also known as Lewy bodies, and they can affect several different regions of the brain. As the proteins build up, surrounding neurons work less effectively, and eventually die.

In Parkinson's disease, Lewy bodies appear primarily in an area of the midbrain called the substantia nigra. This crescent-shaped mass is located just above the spinal cord. In a healthy brain, the cells in the substantia nigra produce and release the chemical dopamine. Dopamine works as a neurotransmitter to send a variety of chemical messages throughout the nervous system. In

## Nutritional Lithium: A Cinderella Story

particular, it works to regulate the reward and addiction centers of the brain, and also helps to coordinate movement and balance. The dopamine produced in the substantia nigra is responsible for sending signals directly to the basal ganglia, a mass of nerve fibers that help to initiate and control movement.

In areas of the brain affected by Parkinson's disease, dopamine production falters. As the unwanted protein "globs" accumulate, the surrounding cells are deprived of nutrients and energy supplies. Without these essential provisions, the cells are no longer able to keep up with the synthesis of dopamine. Soon the neurons begin to die off, and stores of dopamine decrease. Over time, there is not enough dopamine to transmit signals from the midbrain to the spinal cord effectively. This prevents the brain from being able to communicate with the body to synchronize physical activity. Initially, this manifests as sporadic, abnormal movement patterns. As the disease develops further, however, paralysis can occur.

The first sign of Parkinson's disease is usually a subtle tremor of the thumb and forefinger, sometimes called "pill-rolling." Symptoms of the advancing disease vary, but may include:

- Tremor of the hands arms, legs, jaw and face
- Bradykinesia or slowness of movement
- Rigidity and stiffness of the limbs or trunk
- Postural instability or impaired balance and coordination
- Lack of facial expression, difficulty swallowing or speaking

It is important to note that Parkinson's disease itself is not considered fatal. However, complications from the disease are serious; the Centers for Disease Control and Prevention (CDC) rated complications from PD as the 14th top cause of death in the United States (Murphy et al., 2015).

At this time, the causes of Parkinson's are unclear. In about 10% of cases the onset of the disease can be traced to a discrete genetic mutation. In athletes like Muhammad Ali, repeated head trauma is believed to play a significant role. However, the overwhelming majority of Parkinson's cases are deemed idiopathic, meaning that the direct cause is not known. Researchers believe that a complex combination of subtle environmental, biological, and genetic factors can give rise to the disease (Klein & Westenberger, 2012). In other words, the disease results from the interplay of nature and nurture— long-term interactions between genetic make-up, life activities, and environmental exposures (Tanner, 2011).

Currently, the identified risk factors for Parkinson's include:

- Age: typical onset is middle or late life, with vulnerability increasing by years
- Sex: the disease is more common in men than women, although whether this is due to genetics, hormones or differences in behavior is not yet understood
- Toxin Exposure: interaction with pollutants like pesticides and herbicides has been shown to increase disease rate.

## Challenges in Parkinson's Treatment

One of the major difficulties in treating Parkinson's is that symptoms appear late in the disease progression. Oftentimes 60-80% of the neurons in an area of the brain are destroyed before a physical sign appears. This delay makes the disease extremely difficult to detect early on. Once patients present at the doctor's office with clinical symptoms, the internal damage may already be significant—in most cases, too significant to completely reverse.

There is some hope in Parkinson's treatment, however. Various therapies exist to manage symptoms, and many do so quite effectively. A medication called Levodopa has long been considered the gold standard in Parkinson's treatment. Levodopa works by being converted to dopamine in the brain, serving as a replacement for the dopamine that is lost when neurons in the substantia nigra die. When dopamine levels are supplemented in this way, the chemical messaging system between the brain and body is partially restored. Nervous system communication improves, and the characteristic rigidity and tremor associated with Parkinson's subside (NIH, 2015).

# Nutritional Lithium: A Cinderella Story

When it was first introduced nearly 50 years ago, Levodopa revolutionized Parkinson's care. The simple medication provided quick, effective, and much-needed relief from physical manifestations of the illness. However, while Levodopa eases symptoms, it does not shift the underlying course of the disease. Moreover, it is now well documented that most people who take Levodopa develop substantial side effects within 5-10 years of starting on the medicine (Mischley, 2012). These side effects include uncontrollable jerking or twisting movements (otherwise called dyskinesias) that can become as disabling as the disease itself. People may also experience something called the "on-off" effect, wherein Levodopa will work to control symptoms for a time and then randomly and abruptly stop. Affected individuals are thus left to choose between the slowness, rigidity and tremor of Parkinson's or the unpredictable writhing, dyskinetic movements associated with their treatment.

This paradoxical circumstance has left many researchers wondering why there are such unfortunate repercussions to taking a dopamine-replenishing drug like Levodopa. As is the case with most inquiries into the complex and ever-evolving world of neurology, scientists still aren't entirely sure. The prevailing hypothesis to explain this painful dyskinetic response, however, has to do with changes in the sensitivity of dopamine receptors (Thanvi, Lo & Robinson, 2007).

In order to understand this phenomenon, consider how dopamine works in a healthy brain. When a chemical messenger like dopamine is released, it enters a gap between nerve cells that is called a synapse. It crosses this small space and binds to receptors that have been specifically designed for it on the other side. These receptors can be programmed with different levels of sensitivity. When the sensitivity is "high," the receptors detect and pick up more of the neurotransmitter, and when it is "low," they grab up less. The dopamine molecules left in the synapse either remain in this extracellular space or are shuttled back to the releasing neuron.

Researchers believe that what happens with Levodopa and other similar medications is that chronic exposure to this substance increases dopamine receptor sensitivity. At first the transition to the medication is smooth because the receptors are acting normally. Over time, however, the receptors become more sensitive; they are "hungry" and searching for 'real' dopamine. The neurotransmitter is no longer being delivered in a natural, consistent flow; instead it comes in one large rush when the medication is taken and then fades until the next scheduled dose. The receptors become confused and dysfunctional. The pattern of communication between the brain and the body is once again disrupted and movement issues appear.

## Uses of Lithium for Parkinson's Disease

In psychiatry, lithium is commonly used to regulate dopamine activity in disorders where the system is known to be out of control, such as in schizophrenia, ADHD, addiction, and affective disorders. Based on this concept, a couple of researchers hypothesized that lithium salts may work to reduce Levodopa side effects by correcting dopamine receptor super-sensitivity (Dalen & Steg, 1973). If the trial worked, lithium could be used together with Levodopa to prolong its benefits and provide more lasting relief to Parkinson's sufferers.

Researchers selected two individuals suffering from Levodopa side effects whose symptoms were not relieved when the medication dosage was lowered. Lithium was administered to each patient, and they were monitored for two months. In order to reduce the risk of layering on additional adverse effects from the lithium, prescriptions were kept below what is considered the therapeutic dose (serum levels at or below 0.6 mEq/L). During the observation period of the study, both individuals experienced a reduction in Levodopa-induced dyskinesias or tics. The authors concluded that their findings in favor of lithium were positive, but recognized that the small case study design was not sufficient to prove that lithium salts would be useful to remediate Levodopa side effects in Parkinson's patients. Interest in lithium was sparked in the community, and over the next several years an assortment of letters were published in response.

One noteworthy reply appeared in the journal *The Lancet*. A team of researchers shared their results from a similar trail with four Levodopa treated patients who were struggling with dyskinesias. The major difference in this follow-up study was that subjects were prescribed much higher lithium concentrations (450-900 mg) to reach increased blood values of 1.0-1.6 mEq/L. In contrast to the results of the initial study, which found lithium to be very helpful in reducing Levodopa side effects, only a "slight reduction" of uncontrollable tics was reported in two of the four participants in the follow-up. Furthermore, none of the patients involved in this second trial opted to continue lithium after the study period ended. Limited benefits or disruptive side effects including loss of appetite, nausea and sleepiness were cited as the primary reasons to discontinue. From the results of this small, uncontrolled study, the authors were quick to discourage lithium therapy in Parkinson's patients due to concerns over toxicity. (Van Woert and Amandi, 1973). They never considered that the doses they had used, the same doses used in psychiatry to control mania, may simply have been too high.

A more formal piece was released about one year later to provide more substance to this ongoing investigation. Twenty-one Parkinsonian patients were recruited for a single-blind, placebo-controlled trial of lithium carbonate for dyskinesia symptoms. Lithium was started at 250 mg in each participant and then increased until side effects became apparent. Specific lithium blood levels were not reported, but doses were presumably on the high end, or between 900-1200 mg daily. Unsurprisingly, given a target dose sufficient to produce side effects, several participants withdrew due to uncomfortable physical consequences such as unsteadiness, depression, and skin rashes. In those who remained until the study conclusion, no significant improvements in Levodopa-induced dyskinesia were reported (McCaul & Stern, 1974).

Nearly one decade after the initial paper on lithium and Levodopa was published, a study appearing in the *Annals of Neurology* brought lithium back into the discussion of Parkinson's treatment. Six patients with severe Parkinsonism for whom medications had stopped working consistently were treated with lithium carbonate in addition to their regular medications in a randomized double-blind crossover trial. Lithium was individually adjusted to ensure serum levels stayed between 0.6-1.2 mEg/L and no higher. Five of the lithium-treated patients experienced marked reductions in muscle rigidity (akinesia) and an easing of painful dystonic cramps. The resulting improvements in mobility were so striking that responders regained an average of one full grade in Parkinson staging. Benefits were maintained throughout the full 36 weeks of follow-up. In contrast, there was no reported progress during placebo treatment. The authors of the study concluded that "lithium carbonate appears to offer a new and potentially effective approach to treatment" (Coffey et al., 1982).

While previous studies had focused primarily on lithium's uses for ameliorating the tic-like dyskinesia side effects of Levodopa, research was ignoring lithium as a viable treatment to target Parkinson's symptoms directly. A double-blind, placebo-controlled study completed shortly thereafter added to this new string of investigation. A single daily dose of 600 mg slow release lithium was administered to seven patients with disabling dystonia, a type of uncontrollable, sustained muscle contraction that is characteristic of progressing Parkinson's disease. This pharmacological dose was shown to produce therapeutic lithium levels between 0.5-1.2mEq/L. Participants were involved in multiple phases of the study, and alternated between receiving lithium treatment and transitioning to placebo. At the study conclusion researchers reported that painful Parkinsonian cramps were reduced or abolished in the majority of treatment periods with lithium. What's more, these dystonic cramps consistently returned to pretreatment severity between 1-14 days after stopping lithium (Quinn & Marsden, 1986).

## Beyond Dopamine: Lithium & Neuroprotection

Researchers had first become interested in using lithium as an adjunct medication for Parkinson's patients who were suffering with side effects from the drug Levodopa, or for whom anti-Parkinson medications ceased working. Levodopa is known to create a hypersensitivity in dopamine receptors. Lithium, which is a known dopamine agonist, was predicted to modulate this reactivity to restore therapeutic effects. As described above, the results of small, early trials on the topic were mixed. Nonetheless, some evidence did emerge to show that lithium could be helpful for treating Levodopa-induced side effects. Scientists predicted that lithium, when carefully monitored, would be a useful add-on to prolong the benefits of Levodopa and other anti-Parkinson medications.

What many of these early research groups overlooked, however, was that lithium is helpful for Parkinson's in other ways besides minimizing Levodopa-induced side effects. It is well established that lithium works to balance and protect the central nervous system through various mechanisms. Chapter 5 provided a comprehensive overview of the several mechanisms through which lithium works to enhance brain function. When it comes to Parkinson's and other neurogenerative disorders, several neuroprotective actions emerge as most important. Many of the mechanisms below are also relevant to Alzheimer's and dementia.

### *Lithium Suppresses Glycogen Synthase Kinase-3 (GSK3)*

The enzyme Glycogen Synthase Kinase-3 (GSK3) oversees the expression of over forty different proteins in a healthy human body. It interfaces with a number of amino acids to activate, transport, and synthesize the proteins that our cells require for day to day function (Jope & Roh, 2006).

In some neurodegenerative illnesses, such as Alzheimer's disease, GSK3 becomes dysregulated and unwanted proteins accumulate in the brain tissue. A similar pattern occurs in Parkinson's disease, wherein GSK3 spurs the production of alpha-synuclein proteins, the primary substance in Lewy bodies.

Lithium works as a direct GSK3 inhibitor, preventing the over-expression of the enzyme and its target proteins. By inhibiting GSK3, lithium is predicted to stop alpha-synuclein production and slow the formation of Lewy bodies in the substantia nigra and other brain regions (Lauterbach, Fontenelle & Teixeira, 2012).

### *Lithium Promotes Cell Survival*

All cells have a natural waste-removal system that is essential to survival. The process of degrading and recycling cellular debris is called autophagy. In neurodegenerative disorders like Parkinson's disease, the process of autophagy in the neurons can become impaired or disabled. Deposits of abnormal proteins such as alpha-synuclein thus build up in the brain cells more readily and rapidly, leading to dopamine signaling problems, inflammation, and, eventually, neuronal cell death.

Lithium treatment has been shown to restore autophagy in compromised neurons. In other words, lithium ions activate the "garbage disposal" system of

# Lithium as a Medicine: Parkinson's Disease

the cells so that unwanted proteins and other compounds are removed before they become problematic. In animal models, lithium has improved the clearance of intracellular alpha-synuclein from cells, helping slow the formation of Lewy bodies and progression of Parkinson's (Sarkar, et al., 2005; Ravikumar, et al., 2010).

## *LITHIUM DECREASES OXIDATIVE STRESS*

Oxidative stress is believed to be one of the underlying causes of cellular dysfunction and death in Parkinson's. Oxidative stress is essentially an imbalance between the production of free radicals and the ability of the body to counteract their harmful effects through neutralization with antioxidants.

Free radicals are disruptive molecules that are created in the normal course of metabolism, in some disease states, and from burdens in the environment like radiation, toxins in air, food, and water, tobacco smoke and other sources. In Parkinson's sufferers, there is evidence of disproportionately high concentrations of free radicals within the nervous system (Bosco et al., 2006; Nakabeppu et al., 2007). Simultaneously, patients present with abnormally low levels of glutathione, the body's main protective antioxidant. This disparity between high free radical load and low antioxidant defenses creates significant oxidative damage. In Parkinson's the lipids, proteins, and DNA within nerve cells are frequently destroyed by free radicals.

In several in vitro studies, lithium administration was found to protect the cells from this free radical damage (Kim et al., 2011). In addition, lithium has been shown to promote gluathione production, helping to build up defenses against future assaults (de Vasconcellos et al., 2006; Kim et al., 2011). Lithium therefore has a normalizing effect on oxidative stress, which is critical in preventing the nerve cell damage in Parkinson's patients.

## *LITHIUM INCREASES NEUROTROPHIC FACTORS*

Neurotrophins are a family of large proteins that promote the growth and survival of nervous system cells. Because neurotrophins are known to help regulate cell division and growth in neurons, a great deal of research has investigated their therapeutic potential for people suffering from disorders of neuronal degeneration or physical trauma that results in the severing of nerve connections. Increasing the levels of key neurotrophic factors can help direct and facilitate the survival of neurons after injury or in neurodegenerative disease such as Parkinson's disease.

Brain derived neurotrophic factor is one of the key neurotrophic factors in the central nervous system. BDNF is found in the synapses, or spaces, between neurons, where it works to enhance cell-to-cell communication and signaling. There is a growing body of evidence implicating BDNF in the pathogenesis of Parkinson's disease, suggesting that lower levels correlate with increased motor impairment in early stages. Researchers predict that maintaining adequate levels of BDNF would stabilize dopamine signaling and slow disease progression. Raising BDNF levels is thus a key target in the development of neuroprotective therapies for Parkinson's (Scalzo et al., 2010).

Lithium has been found to stimulate the circulation of several key neurotrophic factors, including BDNF (Leyhe et al., 2009; Fukumoto et al., 2001). Not only does chronic lithium therapy increase this key protein at the local or cellular level, but it also optimizes expression of the BDNF *gene*. In patients taking lithium, the gene that codes for BDNF production is left in the "on" position, promoting a consistent release of the protein throughout the nervous system. With this neurotrophic change hardwired at the genetic level, the benefits of BDNF are predicted to be more widespread and longer lasting (Dwivedi & Zhang, 2014).

## Making the Change: Low Dose Lithium for Parkinson's

A growing body of evidence exists to support lithium's neuroprotective qualities. From this research, it is clear that this mineral plays a key role in the central nervous system. Specifically, lithium could have major therapeutic benefits to counteract neurodegeneration in disorders such as Parkinson's disease. Yet, in spite of its exciting potential, lithium has only been tested in small trials and is rarely used in practice for Parkinson's patients. Adverse and bothersome side effects have remained a major stumbling block with treatment. This is especially true for the Parkinson's population, which tends to be older on average and consequently less adept at metabolizing concentrated amounts of lithium.

# Lithium as a Medicine: Parkinson's Disease

Preliminary research has assessed the efficacy of lower doses of lithium in achieving relief from Parkinsonian motor problems. A team led by renowned Parkinson's researcher Julie K. Andersen, PhD recently completed the third in a series of rodent studies on the subject. Mice with a mutation for Parkinson's were treated with an amount of lithium equivalent to about one quarter of what humans would receive for the treatment of psychiatric illness—about one quarter of the amount used in nearly all other trials with lithium for Parkinson's (Lazzara et al., 2015).

Researchers found that low doses of lithium boosted the expression of tyrosine hydroxylase, an enzyme that increases dopamine synthesis. When asked to describe the effects, Andersen stated, "We clearly saw a prevention of the motor difficulties we would expect to see in the animals. The treatment also protected the area of the brain that is normally damaged by Parkinson's" (Buck Institute, 2015).

Andersen's enthusiasm about low dose lithium is unmistakable. In 2012 she co-filed an application for a patent entitled "Low Dose Lithium in the Treatment or Prophylaxis of Parkinson's Disease," laying claim to all forms, physiologic doses, and strategies of augmentation for this naturally occurring mineral, alone or in combination with other interventions in the treatment of Parkinson's. The patent states that the chronic administration of low dose lithium may be used to inhibit the onset of progression or lessen the severity of Parkinson's symptoms (Andersen & Kim, 2012).

Other researchers such as Laurie K. Mischley, ND, MPG, PhD have been equally enthusiastic about the neuroprotective potential of low or trace-dose lithium. Mischley's main interest lies in determining whether lithium deficiency may be a contributing factor to growing rates of neurodegenerative illnesses like Parkinson's. Studies are underway to investigate the prevalence of lithium deficiency in this population (Mischley, 2014).

There is urgent need for more research on low dose lithium in the treatment of Parkinson's. In an institutional press release about the findings of Anderson's most current study, David K. Simon, MD, PhD, Associate Professor of Neurology at Harvard Medical School in Boston and chair of the Scientific Review Committee for the Parkinson's Study Group, a not-for-profit network of Parkinson's Centers, stated: "this study provides additional evidence on top of prior work from Dr. Andersen's lab and others that lithium may have therapeutic potential in Parkinson's disease, which is a hypothesis that should be tested in clinical trials" (Buck Institute, 2015).

## Potential Relief for Parkinson's Disease with Lithium

Parkinson's disease is a disorder of the central nervous system that affects motor movement. Tremors, rigidity, muscles stiffness, and postural instability are among the primary symptoms. Movement issues manifest from the uncontrolled death of dopamine-generating cells in the substantia nigra, an area of the midbrain that controls movement.

Parkinson's is a chronic and progressive illness for which there are limited treatment options, but no cure. Levodopa has long been the only medication available for Parkinson's therapy. Levodopa is converted into dopamine in the brain, serving as a replacement for the natural dopamine that is lost when neurons in the substantia nigra die. This medication can reduce symptoms and can improve the quality of life for some Parkinson's patients. Unfortunately, Levodopa doesn't work effectively as a long-term treatment. Eventually it creates further problems with dopamine exchange in the brain, resulting in side effects that can be as debilitating as Parkinson's itself. Lithium is a viable option for counterbalancing this issue. It is our hope that future studies work to find this answer.

## CHAPTER 8 | References

Andersen, J.K & Kim, H. (2013). *U.S. Patent No. 0017274*. Novato, CA: U.S. Patent and Trademark Office.

Bosco, D. A., Fowler, D. M., Zhang, Q., Nieva, J., Powers, E. T., Wentworth, P. J., & ... Kelly, J. W. (2006). Elevated levels of oxidized cholesterol metabolites in Lewy body disease brains accelerate alpha-synuclein fibrilization. *Nature Chemical Biology, 2*(5), 249-253.

Buck Institute. (2015). *Low dose lithium reduces side effects from most common treatment for Parkinson's disease*. Retrieved from www.buckinstitute.org/buck-news/low-dose-lithium-reduces-side-effects-most-common-treatment-parkinsons-disease

Coffey, C. E., Ross, D. R., Ferren, E. L., Sullivan, J. L., & Olanow, C. W. (1982). Treatment of the "on-off" phenomenon in Parkinsonism with lithium carbonate. *Annals of Neurology, 12*(4), 375-379.

Dalén, P., & Steg, G. (1973). Lithium and levodopa in parkinsonism. *Lancet, 1*(7809), 936-937.

de Vasconcellos, A. S., Nieto, F. B., Crema, L. M., Diehl, L. A., de Almeida, L. M., Prediger, M. E., & ... Dalmaz, C. (2006). Chronic lithium treatment has antioxidant properties but does not prevent oxidative damage induced by chronic variate stress. *Neurochemical Research, 31*(9), 1141-1151.

Dwivedi, T., & Zhang, H. (2015). Lithium-induced neuroprotection is associated with epigenetic modification of specific BDNF gene promoter and altered expression of apoptotic-regulatory proteins. *Frontiers in Neuroscience, 8*, 457.

Fukumoto, T., Morinobu, S., Okamoto, Y., Kagaya, A., & Yamawaki, S. (2001). Chronic lithium treatment increases the expression of brain-derived neurotrophic factor in the rat brain. *Psychopharmacology, 158*(1), 100-106.

Jope, R. S., & Roh, M. (2006). Glycogen synthase kinase-3 (GSK3) in psychiatric diseases and therapeutic interventions. *Current Drug Targets, 7*(11), 1421-1434.

Kim, Y., Rane, A., Lussier, S., & Andersen, J. K. (2011). Lithium protects against oxidative stress-mediated cell death in α-synuclein-overexpressing in vitro and in vivo models of Parkinson's disease. *Journal of Neuroscience Research, 89*(10), 1666-1675.

Klein, C. & Westenberfer, A. (2012). Genetics of Parkinson's disease. *Cold Spring Harbor Perspectives in Medicine, 2*(1), a008888.

Kowal, S. L., Dall, T. M., Chakrabarti, R., Storm, M. V., & Jain, A. (2013). The current and projected economic burden of Parkinson's disease in the United States. *Movement Disorders, 28*(3), 311-318.

Lauterbach, E. C., Fontenelle, L. F., & Teixeira, A. L. (2012). The neuroprotective disease-modifying potential of psychotropics in Parkinson's disease. *Parkinson's Disease, 2012,* 753548.

Lazzara, C. A., & Yong-Hwan, K. (2015). Potential application of lithium in Parkinson's and other neurodegenerative diseases. *Frontiers in Neuroscience, 9,* 403.

Lazzara, C. A., Riley, R. R., Rane, A., Andersen, J. K., & Kim, Y. (2015). The combination of lithium and l-Dopa/Carbidopa reduces MPTP-induced abnormal involuntary movements (AIMs) via calpain-1 inhibition in a mouse model: Relevance for Parkinson's disease therapy. *Brain Research, 1622,* 127-136.

Leyhe, T., Eschweiler, G. W., Stransky, E., Gasser, T., Annas, P., Basun, H., & Laske, C. (2009). Increase of BDNF serum concentration in lithium treated patients with early Alzheimer's disease. *Journal of Alzheimer's Disease, 16*(3), 649-656.

McCaul, J. A., & Stern, G. M. (1974). Letter: Lithium in Parkinson's disease. *Lancet, 1*(7866), 1117.

Mischley, L. (2012). Lithium deficiency in Parkinson's disease. University of Washington MPH thesis. Unpublished.

Mischley, L. (2014). The Role of Lithium in Neurological Health and Disease. *Journal of Orthomolecular Medicine, 29*(3), 101.

Murphy, L. et al. (2015). Deaths: Final data for 2012. *Centers for Disease Control National Vital Statistics Reports, 63*(9), 1-118.

Nakabeppu, Y., Tsuchimoto, D., Yamaguchi, H., & Sakumi, K. (2007). Oxidative damage in nucleic acids and Parkinson's disease. *Journal of Neuroscience Research, 85*(5), 919-934.

National Institutes of Health (NIH). (2015). *Levodopa and Carbidopa.* MedlinePlus. Retrieved from www.nlm.nih.gov/medlineplus/druginfo/meds/a601068.html

Quinn, N. & Marsden, C. D. (1986). Lithium for painful dystonia in Parkinson's disease. *Lancet, 1*(8494), 1377.

Ravikumar, B., Sarkar, S., Davies, J. E., Futter, M., Garcia-Arencibia, M., Green-Thompson, Z. W., & ... Rubinsztein, D. C. (2010). Regulation of mammalian autophagy in physiology and pathophysiology. *Physiological Reviews, 90*(4), 1383-435.

Scalzo, P., Kummer, A., Bretas, T. L., Cardoso, F., & Teixeira, A. L. (2010). Serum levels of brain-derived neurotrophic factor correlate with motor impairment in Parkinson's disease. *Journal of Neurology, 257*(4), 540.

Sarkar, S., Floto, R. A., Berger, Z., Imarisio, S., Cordenier, A., Pasco, M., & ... Rubinsztein, D. C. (2005). Lithium Induces Autophagy by Inhibiting Inositol Monophosphatase. *Journal of Cell Biology, 170*(7), 1101-11.

Tanner, C. M. (2011). Environmental factors and Parkinson's: What have we learned? *Parkinson's Disease Foundation Newsletter.* Spring 2011.

Thanvi, B., Lo, N., & Robinson, T. (2007). Levodopa-induced dyskinesia in Parkinson's disease: clinical features, pathogenesis, prevention and treatment. *Postgraduate Medical Journal, 83*(980), 384-388.

Van Woert, M. H., & Ambani, L. M. (1973). Lithium and levodopa in parkinsonism. *Lancet, 1*(7816), 1390-1391.

# Nine

## LITHIUM AS A MEDICINE: MOOD DISORDERS

"Mainstay." "Gold Standard." "Benchmark." "First-line." "Best tolerated." "Hallmark." These words of praise have all been used to describe the role of lithium in the treatment of mood disorders.

Lithium has long been known to have mood-balancing effects. As early as Ancient Greek and Roman times, people were advised to soak in alkali-rich mineral springs to soothe "meloncholia" and "mania." In the mid-1800s, pharmacological amounts of lithium were being used as a treatment for acute mania at New York's Bellevue Hospital Medical Center. In the 1940's, Australian Psychiatrist John Cade began experiencing great successes using the carbonate form of lithium as a treatment for manic depression. By the time lithium received FDA approval for the treatment of mood disorders in the 1970's, a great deal of evidence already existed to show that it had powerful nervous system stabilizing effects.

Since then scientific knowledge about the efficacy of lithium in treating mood disorders has only continued to grow. Study after study has been published to establish lithium as the most successful treatment option for patients with bipolar disorder and refractory major depression. However, while papers in praise of lithium pile up, clinical use has been on a slow decline. Fears over the toxic potential of high-dose lithium and the tedium of needing to closely monitor serum levels in patients taking the medication have made it somewhat cumbersome to use in modern clinical practice. Insufficient training of psychiatrists in the use of lithium therapy and the aggressive marketing of alternative medications are also likely to blame for the downtrend in use (Young & Hammond, 2007).

A new wave in research is looking to revive lithium therapy by going back to its ancient roots. Evidence is gradually accumulating to show that low doses of lithium, doses found naturally in groundwater, may have profound mood-balancing effects. While it may seem improbable the small amounts of this mineral could have an impact on mood, the more researchers look, the more they seem to find. Lithium continues to hold valuable potential for patients with mood disorders and for the providers treating them.

## A Closer Look at Mood Disorders

Mood disorders, also called affective disorders, are a category of illnesses that involve a serious change in underlying emotional state. The two most common types of mood disorders are depression and bipolar disorder.

### *Depression*

Depression is the leading cause of disability worldwide in terms of total years lost due to illness. Best estimates state that between 5-20% of us will experience a major depressive episode at some point in our lives, leading to hospitalization, intensive therapy, or treatment with pharmaceuticals (WHO, 2015).

Depression is different from the day-to-day "blues" or emotional responses we have to problems we may encounter. Feeling sad or upset after a traumatic life event is expected and not a cause for concern. However, when extreme sadness settles in for no concrete reason or feelings of intense desolation persist for a prolonged period of time, depression may be the cause.

Depression is a neurological disorder manifesting as low mood, decreased energy, and feelings of low self-worth. The disorder involves severe symptoms that interfere with one's ability to work, sleep, study, eat, and enjoy life.

Symptoms of depression include:

- Changes in sleep - trouble falling asleep, staying asleep or sleeping much longer than usual
- Changes in appetite - leading to weight changes when a person stops eating or uses food as a coping mechanism
- Lack of concentration – difficulty making decisions
- Loss of energy - feeling fatigue, thinking slowly or being unable to perform normal daily routines
- Lack of interest in usual activities or loss of capacity to experience pleasure
- Low self-esteem - dwelling on losses or failures and feeling excessive guilt
- Hopelessness - feeling that nothing good will ever happen
- Physical aches and pains

## *Bipolar Disorder*

Bipolar disorder, also known as manic-depressive disorder, involves dramatic fluctuations between manic highs and depressive lows. In other words, individuals with bipolar disorder experience periods in which they feel euphoric and energized, and other times in which they are extremely hopeless and sad. In between these periods, individuals generally feel normal. You can think of these highs and lows as the two "poles" of mood, which is why it's called "bipolar" disorder. This contrasts with unipolar depression (or what we tend to simply call depression) as discussed above, which involves only periods of low mood.

People with bipolar disorder are more likely to seek help when they are depressed than when experiencing manic symptoms (Hirschfield, 2005). Thus, a careful medical history is needed to assure that bipolar disorder is not mistakenly diagnosed as depression.

Symptoms of mania or a manic episode include:

- Elevated mood: prolonged period of feeling "high" or overly happy.
- Extreme irritability: easily distracted, restless, upset.

- Behaving impulsively: engaging in pleasurable, high-risk behaviors.
- Lack of sleep: not feeling tired.
- Racing thoughts: pressured speech; speaking rapidly, and jumping from one idea to another

Symptoms of a depressive episode include:

- Low mood: extended sadness or hopelessness
- Fatigue: feeling tired and slowed down
- Loss of interest: no desire to engage in activities that were once enjoyed
- Trouble concentrating: inability to focus, remember or make decisions

## Determining a Cause

Mood disorders do not have one discrete cause. The illnesses are instead believed to arise from the interplay of genetic and biological factors with life experiences. Trauma, loss of a loved one, job loss, a difficult relationship, or any stressful situation may trigger a depressive episode; however, an obvious precipitating factor is not always present.

Those who have an immediate family member with a mood disorder are two to three times more likely to develop some form of depression, suggesting that there is a genetic component at play. Technological advances are improving genetic research in the field of mood disorders, although studying this area has proven difficult. The Bipolar Disorder Phenome Database was recently launched to provide an organized repository for documenting and linking visible mood disorder signs with the genes that influence them (Potash, 2007).

Neuroimaging studies have allowed researchers to observe that those who suffer from mood disorders have brains that look and function differently than those who do not suffer from depression. Studies have shown that the frontal lobe of the brain becomes less active when a person is depressed. Changes are seen most dramatically in the prefrontal cortex, which is the center for planning advanced cognitive behavior, expressing personality, and moderating social behavior. The hippocampus, an area of the brain that acts as a gateway between memory and mood, also appears smaller and weaker with depressive illness. Meanwhile the amygdala, the structure where emotional memories are stored, can become more active, especially when episodes are recurrent and there is some kind of trauma involved in the etiology (Gotlib & Hamilton, 2008).

There is also some evidence to show that the process of brain development and growth in early life can have an influence on mood disorder symptoms. For example, one study using MRI found that the pattern of brain development in children with bipolar disorder was similar to that in children with "multi-dimensional impairment," a disorder that causes symptoms that overlap somewhat with bipolar disorder and schizophrenia. This suggests that the pattern of brain development in the two conditions may be associated with the risk for unstable moods (Gogtay, 2007).

At a biochemical level, there appears to be a strong relationship between abnormal levels of neurotransmitters, the substances in our brain that affect mood, and clinical depression. Some people who are depressed have low levels of neurotransmitters like serotonin, dopamine and norepinephrine. In such cases antidepressants can work to increase the level of these chemicals in the brain and help relieve depressive symptoms. On the other hand, it has been shown that others struggling with depression have *low* levels of neurotransmitters (Nutt, 2009). The exact link between depressive symptoms and neurotransmitters is therefore not clearly understood and it is still not known whether changes in levels of neurotransmitters cause the development of depression or if depression causes the changes in neurotransmitters.

Multiple studies have also linked depression with increased markers of inflammation in the body. Inflammation occurs as a result of imbalances between pro-inflammatory mediators and anti-inflammatory mediators. The role of inflammation in Major Depressive Disorder (MDD) has been studied over the past two decades and it is now known that MDD involves both immune suppression as well as immune activation (Blume et al., 2011). Cytokines are small proteins that are released by cells for communication in immune responses. In one study, there were striking similarities between the symptoms of cytokine-induced sickness behavior and depression including anorexia, weight loss, anhedonia, anxiety, and neurocognitive symptoms (Maes et al., 2012).

## Lithium as a Medicine: Mood Disorders

Two large analyses from 2010 and 2012 collectively reviewed data from 53 studies, as well as several postmortem studies, and found that people with depression had signs of widespread inflammation in the brain and other organs (Dowlati, 2010; Liu, Ho & Mak, 2012). Related research has confirmed that inflammation-causing conditions, such as autoimmune disorders and infections, greatly increase risk for developing a mood disorder. A Danish study published in *JAMA Psychiatry* looked at the medical records of over 3 million people and found that a history of infection was associated with a 62% increase in risk of later developing depression or bipolar disorder. The same paper found that a past autoimmune disorder raised risk by 45% (Benros et al., 2013).

Recent research has found that lithium may protect the brain from neuroinflammation, a process whereby sensitive brain cells can become easily damaged (Basselin et al., 2010). In one study, mice were either fed a diet containing lithium chloride or a diet free of lithium for six weeks. At the end the study, researchers introduced inflammation-inducing bacteria and analyzed levels of inflammatory markers in the brain. The researchers found that the group supplemented with lithium had reduced levels of the inflammatory compound arachidonic acid and increased levels of the anti-inflammatory compound 17-hydroxy-docosahexaenoic acid (17-OH-DHA).

While intriguing, the research for the most part has only revealed associations between inflammation and mental health issues; cause and effect has yet to be proven. Nonetheless, the immune system seems to be an important area to consider when looking at the complex pathophysiology of these disorders and appropriate treatment.

All of these diverse mechanisms come into play when considering treatment strategies for individuals with mood disorders.

## Challenges in Treatment

Although there are established treatments for depression, fewer than half of depressed individuals receive treatment. In some countries, only 10% receive treatment. Lack of financial resources, stigma around mental disorders, and inaccurate diagnoses are some barriers to receiving effective care (WHO,

2015). For those who do receive care, the most common treatments are medication and psychotherapy.

The most popular medication choice for treating depressive symptoms is antidepressants such as fluoxetine (Prozac), paroxetine (Paxil) and sertraline (Zoloft). Antidepressant medications work by balancing neurotransmitters, such as serotonin, norepinephrine, and dopamine. Unfortunately, antidepressant medications do not work for everyone; in practice, 50-66% of patients with depression will not recover fully on an antidepressant medication (Gaynes et al., 2008). The most common side effects are headache, nausea, sleeplessness or drowsiness, and agitation. Paradoxically, the FDA also requires a warning on all antidepressant medications stating that there is an increased risk of suicidal thinking or attempts in children, adolescents, and young adults up through age 24. This is troublesome, especially since the medications are designed to be administered to a population already vulnerable to such dangerous symptoms.

For bipolar patients, taking an antidepressant alone can increase the risk of switching to mania, or of developing rapid-cycling symptoms (Thase & Sachs, 2000). For this reason, antidepressants are avoided or more commonly prescribed in combination with a mood-stabilizer like lithium, or an anticonvulsant or antipsychotic medication.

People with depression that has not responded to medication or psychotherapy may turn to brain stimulation therapies. During this type of therapy, specific areas of the brain are stimulated with electricity or magnetic fields. The procedures can cause side effects, including memory loss. In general, the earlier treatment begins, the more effective the outcomes.

Thus, while there are many anti-depressive treatments available today, a disproportionate few seem to respond well to them over the long term. Rates of relapse in depression hover around a disappointing 50%, with affected individuals experiencing an average of five to nine incapacitating depressive episodes over their lifetimes. Now, as more and more individuals present with symptoms, the need for effective and rapidly working treatment strategies has become more pressing than ever.

One well-documented but underused therapy is the mineral lithium.

## History of Lithium and Bipolar Depression

Since its induction into modern psychiatry in 1949, lithium has long been considered the benchmark treatment for managing bipolar illness. It has been extensively used and studied for over sixty years and has been shown in countless trials to help manage acute episodes of mania. Although some of the earlier historic trials have been scrutinized for methodological flaws, lithium's therapeutic value has continued to shine through in modern research. A recent review spanning three decades of solid data affirmed lithium's superior clinical effectiveness for treating the manic phase of bipolar disorder (Baldessarini & Tondo, 2000). Beneficial effects from lithium are predicted to appear in approximately 60–80% of bipolar patients, with no tolerance or sensitivity developing throughout many years when treatment is properly managed (Lepkifker, et al., 2007).

It is in this context of long-term maintenance and prophylaxis that lithium is thought to most powerfully outperform other drugs. Newer pharmaceutical formulations have shown promise in managing acute bipolar mania, for example, but none have matched lithium in long-term effectiveness. This is important, as there is a marked tendency of manic episodes to repeat. It has been estimated that at least 80% of patients who have an episode of mania will have one or more recurrences (NIMH/NIH, 1985; 2002). In a meta-analysis reviewing data from 1,580 bipolar patients, lithium was found to be superior to other common classes of drugs in the prevention of manic episodes (Severus et al., 2014). A different meta-analysis looking at 14 randomized control trials of various mood stabilizers found that lithium had a similar prophylactic influence on depressive cycles as well (Smith, 2007). In a review of observational, naturalistic studies presented at the European Psychiatric Association (EPA) 23rd Congress, a group of researchers released their conclusion that lithium continues to outshine the latest atypical antipsychotics, antidepressants and anti-convulsants in long-term treatment for bipolar disorder. Session moderator Birgit Völlm, MD, PhD, wrapped things up by stating, "Lithium is still the best one" (Simhandl, 2015).

Lithium toxicity, a consequence of poorly managed lithium therapy, has remained a very real concern for many providers. The phenomenon was comprehensively described in a systematic review in 2012. The authors reviewed

385 studies on the subject and concluded that among individuals with mood disorders treated with pharmacological doses of lithium, there was an increased risk of reduced urinary concentrating ability, hypothyroidism, hyperparathyroidism and weight gain (McKnight et al., 2012). Adverse effects, however, are considered to arise much more frequently when serum concentrations are above what is considered within the "therapeutic range." Thus, close monitoring and dose managing are needed to prevent side effects and toxicity, but with this oversight, lithium therapy can be effective and safe. Lithium has been called the only "true" mood stabilizer and has remained a mainstay in bipolar treatment for over half a century (Malhi, 2007).

Less attention has been paid to lithium's potential to treat and prevent unipolar depression, although the literature on the subject is abundant. Research looking into lithium's antidepressant qualities began as early as the 1950s, when researchers started to assess how bipolar patients in the depressive phase responded to lithium. Substantial data was collected to suggest that lithium had stand-alone antidepressant qualities, in addition to its mood stabilizing capabilities. A meta-analysis of studies conducted since this time has indicated that lithium is indeed superior to placebo across a range of plasma levels and dosages for both treating and preventing relapse in depressive patients (Souza & Goodwin, 1991). Another comprehensive review of studies conducted between the years 1950 and 2006 confirmed that lithium effectively prevents the recurrence of unipolar depression across patient groups (Davis et al., 2006).

## Lithium as an Augmentation Therapy

A new use for lithium in the treatment of depression emerged in the 1980s: lower-doses of lithium salts as an augmentation therapy. Patients who respond only partially to antidepressant drugs are typically presented with two options: switch to a new medication or add a second drug to enhance, or augment, treatment. One advantage of augmentation is that it eliminates the period of transition from one medication to another. Secondly, when augmentation works well, it can have a rapidly acting effect.

# Lithium as a Medicine: Mood Disorders

The first study to test the use of lithium as an augmenting agent was conducted by De Montigny and colleagues in 1981. In eight patients who had not responded to at least 3 weeks of treatment with tricyclic antidepressants, a dramatic improvement was seen within 48 hours of the addition of lithium. Subsequent randomized control trials have confirmed these initial findings with more than 30 open-label and comparator studies including more than 500 depressed patients (Bauer et al., 2003, 2010). In these studies lithium was used to augment antidepressant medications of many different kinds, including selective serotonin repute inhibitors (SSRIs), tri- and tetra-cyclic antidepressants and mono-amine oxidase inhibitors. Lithium was found to complement each variety to some extent, with a median response rate of about 56%.

Another meta-analysis of lithium augmentation pooled 10 randomized, double-blind, placebo-controlled studies on the subject (Crossley & Bauer, 2007). This type of placebo-controlled trial is considered the gold standard in today's research practices, and thus the results from this more recent meta-analysis have been highly regarded. The analysis found, after reviewing results from 269 patients mainly with unipolar depression, that lithium had a significant positive effect versus placebo. The few trials in the pooling that had negative findings were predicted to have had too short a duration of treatment, too few participants, or to have used a drug that didn't pair well with lithium. It will thus be important in future research to determine exactly how much and how long lithium should be used in order to achieve optimal results. It will be interesting to see if low dose lithium proves effective in this realm.

It has been argued that lithium is the best-evidenced augmentation therapy in the treatment of depressed patients who do not find improvement with standard anti-depressants. However, the question remains as to whether a positive response to lithium augmentation is indicative of a true synergistic effect with certain medications, or whether the improvements are simply due to the antidepressant effect of lithium on its own. It is also unclear as to what dose and treatment duration works best. Either way, decades of literature have made it abundantly clear that lithium has tremendous potential as an antidepressant therapy—a potential that has been left largely untapped in clinical practice.

# Nutritional Lithium: A Cinderella Story

## Key Mechanisms

Three factors have been identified as key predictors of lithium's effectiveness as an antidepressant: presence of bipolar disorder, high frequency of major depressive episodes, and a family history of major depressive disorder/bipolar disorder in a first-degree relative (Sugawara et al., 2010). These findings suggest that lithium's mood-stabilizing and antidepressant qualities are closely related, and also hint that the mechanisms involved are likely related to genetic or epigenetic changes. Yet despite years of research, it is still unclear *exactly* how lithium works within the cells to provide relief from depressive symptoms.

Several hypotheses currently exist to explain the underlying actions behind the mineral's antidepressant and mood-stabilizing effects.

### *Lithium Augments Serotonergic System*

One popular theory that is currently used to explain the pathological cause of depression is the monoamine hypothesis, as described earlier in this chapter. This theory suggests that mood disorders are linked to dysfunctional serotonin and/or norepinephrine neurotransmission. The hypothesis has been supported by the finding that most antidepressants help to optimize the relay of these chemicals throughout the brain, especially the serotonergic actions.

From human studies we know that lithium has a generally net-enhancing effect on serotonin, meaning it optimizes the amount available for use in the brain and across other systems in the body such as the digestive system (Chenu & Bourin, 2006; Bschor et al, 2002, 2003). Animal studies have provided a deeper understanding of how this occurs, and have shown that lithium works to support and balance the serotonergic system in a multitude of ways (Wegener et al, 2003). For example, lithium ions may repair problems with the synthesis, uptake, storage, release, and/or catabolism of the neurotransmitter to ensure that there is an appropriate amount available to the cells. Some studies have even suggested that lithium improves the operation of the serotonin receptors as well, which help to grab up the important chemical so that it can be properly used by the cells (Price, 1990). Clearly, lithium does not simply increase or decrease serotonin levels, but also helps to regulate its transport throughout the nervous system.

# Lithium as a Medicine: Mood Disorders

### *LITHIUM WORKS ON GLYCOGEN SYNTHASE KINASE-3 (GSK3)*
The enzyme Glycogen synthase kinase-3, often shortened to GSK3, has a strong influence on neuronal function, structure, remodeling, cell survival, and gene expression. It is also deeply intertwined with the activity of several important neurotransmitter groups, including the serotonergic, dopaminergic, cholinergic, and glutamatergic systems. Increasing research studies identify that problems with GSK3 are also involved in the development and progression of mood disorders, including bipolar disorder and major depression.

Investigation of the link between GSK3 and mood disorders first began in 1996 with the discovery that lithium directly inhibits the enzyme. Researchers hypothesized at this time that lithium's mood-stabilizing and antidepressant effects may in fact be the result of the mineral's ability to regulate this enzyme (Klein & Melton, 1996). Additional evidence has accumulated to support this hypothesis, showing that GSK3 is often hyperactive in individuals struggling with depressive symptoms. Given these findings, GSK3 has become a key therapeutic target for affective disorders research (Jope & Roh, 2006). Other mood stabilizers have been shown to inhibit GSK3 as well, but none have been found to do so to the same extent as lithium. Valproic acid, for example, which was originally used as an anticonvulsant and is now widely used as a mood stabilizer in bipolar disorder, has been reported by some investigators but not by others to directly inhibit GSK3 activity. The GSK3 theory could possibly explain why lithium has remained successful both in treating mood disorders independently and when coupled with antidepressants that work on similar neurotransmitter systems.

### *LITHIUM INCREASES GRAY MATTER IN THE BRAIN*
With technological advances, scientists have clearly established that depressed brains look different from healthy ones. One trait frequently seen in those with depression is a shrinking of gray matter—the type of brain tissue that contains all of the nerve cell bodies. This shrinking of tissue is most prominent in areas of the brain that help with emotional regulation. Scientists aren't entirely sure how or why this tissue loss happens, but there is evidence to show that reversing the process can improve depressive symptoms.

Using Magnetic Resonance Imaging or MRI technology to take "pictures" of the brain, researchers have discovered that patients taking lithium show increases in gray matter over time (Kempton, 2008). This happens most dramatically in the hippocampus, an area that is vital for storing memories and emotions. It is thought that lithium ions help to regenerate nerve cells in this area, thus helping the brain recover its normal emotional functioning. This neuro-regenerative phenomenon has profound implications for treating affective disorders and other neurological conditions.

### *LITHIUM PROTECTS AGAINST INFLAMMATION*

In acute situations, inflammation is a natural, protective process. It is an innate response by the immune system to deliver white blood cells and other healing factors to areas of tissue that are injured or damaged in some way. In the nervous system, inflammation helps stimulate repair and recovery of compromised neurons. However, if inflammation in the nervous system or other areas of the body continues well after the immediate injury or threat is over, it can become widespread and very damaging. This type of unchecked inflammation is associated with mental health symptoms, including depression and mania.

A recent meta-analysis of 29 studies confirmed that patients with depression have elevated levels of pro-inflammatory chemicals called cytokines (Liu, Ho & Mak, 2012). Cytokines are the messenger molecules of the immune system and include a diverse assortment of compounds called interleukins, interferons, and growth factors. Lithium helps to moderate inflammation by dampening cytokine reactivity. In particular, it reduces the production of two pro-inflammatory cytokines known as interleukin-1B and tumor necrosis factor (Boufidou et al. 2004, Nahman, 2012).

## Low Dose Lithium for Depression

All evidence considered, lithium is one of the most extensively studied but underused therapies available for the treatment of depression. Although lithium is most widely known for its ability to stabilize the fluctuating high and

## Lithium as a Medicine: Mood Disorders

low moods seen in bipolar disorder, it has also proven valuable for treating and preventing unipolar depression. Over sixty years of research and clinical evidence exist to demonstrate that lithium can be a safe and effective antidepressant therapy at a range of doses. More recent studies have suggested that lithium can be helpful in combination with other antidepressant medications to augment therapeutic benefits and increase chances of treatment success.

Although how exactly lithium works within the body to relieve depressive symptoms remains unclear, several hypotheses exist. There is significant evidence to show that lithium helps to balance levels of the neurotransmitter serotonin and to aid in its circulation throughout the nervous system. Other studies have demonstrated that lithium inhibits the enzyme GSK3, which is thought to become hyperactive in those with mood disorders. Downstream, this enzyme also works to enhance neurotransmission throughout the brain and body, and is thus thought to directly impact mood. Lithium also decreases inflammation in the brain and other organs, helping to improve depressive symptoms.

Therefore,with this impressive body of research available to support lithium's use as an antidepressant and mood stabilizer, it seems strange that the mineral's popularity is declining in clinical settings (Fenn et al, 1996; Blanco et al, 2002). There seems to be no remarkable explanation for this discrepancy, although we suppose several factors play a part. First, lithium does carry with it great deal of stigma from its long history in psychiatry and use in the management of severe mental illness. Secondly, lithium is also an old drug with no commercial champion to promote it. Without vested interest, lithium has become lost in the barrage of lucrative new antidepressants that hit the market every year. Lastly, some providers may be hesitant to prescribe lithium at high doses due to the monitoring that is required to prevent side effects. We believe that low dose lithium, or lithium used in amounts more closely mimicking those found in food and water, could resolve this last concern.

In pharmacotherapy, lithium doses tend to range from 900-2400 mg/day for an individual to obtain serum levels of 0.6 to 1.5 mEq/L. Paradoxically, little literature exists to support appropriate targets for lithium intake, either among healthy individuals or those with mental health disorders (Mischley,

2014). Most studies focus on the toxic effects of too much lithium in the system, while a lower limit has not been sufficiently explored.

The mood-enhancing properties of natural lithium have been promoted for hundreds (if not thousands) of years- well before pharmacological lithium tablets hit the market. The Bohemian spas in the Czech Republic were among the most famous of the historic European springs rumored to improve mood and well-being in those choosing to bathe in them. Dr. Schrauzer, then a chemist at a local research institute specializing in mineral waters, analyzed these springs in 1948. He found the waters had unusually high lithium concentration compared to other springs in the area. His unpublished data led Dr. Schrauzer, now Professor Emeritus in the Department of Chemistry and Biochemistry at the University of California, San Diego, to continue throughout his career the study of the nutritional essentiality of lithium in mood (Mischley, 2014). Most notably, his research has spurred a recent series of 11 ecological studies that have linked low lithium concentrations in tap water with adverse behavioral, legal, and medical outcomes (Kapusta & Konig, 2015).

Unfortunately, only one intervention study of nutritional lithium has been published. In 1994, 24 former drug users were randomized to receive either 400 micrograms of lithium, or placebo, for four weeks in an attempt to evaluate whether lithium improved mood. In the lithium group, there was a statistically significant improvement in week four mood scores from baseline, specifically on scales for happiness, friendliness, and energy. These changes were not seen in the placebo group (Schrauzer & deVroey, 1994).

Although few trials exist that show how low dose lithium can improve mood, there is ample evidence to show that the nutrient has neuroprotective and balancing effects in the central nervous system. We have hundreds of case studies from our practice to suggest that nutritional lithium has an important part to play in the treatment of mood disorders. Clinical experience coupled with multiple epidemiological studies connecting low lithium levels in drinking water with higher rates of psychiatric illness, certainly provide a strong foundation for further exploration. Additional research into the effects of low dose lithium for mood disorders is warranted.

# Lithium as a Medicine: Mood Disorders

Global rates of mood disorders are on the rise, and there is a pressing need for safe, targeted interventions to resolve devastating mood disorders. In recent years the number of pharmacological agents available for treating patients with mood disorders has surged, but lithium remains one of the best-tolerated treatment options for many patients. Given this evidence, psychiatrists should continue to include this time-tested therapy in their arsenal for treating depression and consider the potential of adjunctive nutritional lithium.

## CHAPTER 9 | References

Baldessarini, R. J., & Tondo, L. (2000). Does lithium treatment still work? Evidence of stable responses over three decades. *Archives of General Psychiatry, 57*(2), 187-190.

Basselin, M., Kim, H., Chen, M., Ma, K., Rapoport, S. I., Murphy, R. C., & Farias, S. E. (2010). Lithium modifies brain arachidonic and docosahexaenoic metabolism in rat lipopolysaccharide model of neuroinflammation. *Journal of Lipid Research, 51*(5), 1049-1056.

Bauer, M., Adli, M., Baethge, C., Berghöfer, A., Sasse, J., Heinz, A., & Bschor, T. (2003). Lithium augmentation therapy in refractory depression: Clinical evidence and neurobiological mechanisms. *Canadian Journal of Psychiatry, 48*(7), 440-446.

Bauer, M., Adli, M., Bschor, T., Pilhatsch, M., Pfennig, A., Sasse, J., & ... Lewitzka, U. (2010). Lithium's emerging role in the treatment of refractory major depressive episodes: Augmentation of antidepressants. *Neuropsychobiology, 62*(1), 36-42.

Benros, M. E., Waltoft, B. L., Nordentoft, M., Østergaard, S. D., Eaton, W. W., Krogh, J., & Mortensen, P. B. (2013). Autoimmune diseases and severe infections as risk factors for mood disorders: A nationwide study. *JAMA Psychiatry, 70*(8), 812-820.

Blanco, C., Laje, G., Olfson, M., Marcus, S. C., & Pincus, H. A. (2002). Trends in the treatment of bipolar disorder by outpatient psychiatrists. *American Journal of Psychiatry, 159*(6). 1005.

Blume, J., Douglas, S. D., & Evans, D. L. (2011). Immune suppression and immune activation in depression. *Brain Behavior and Immunity, 25*(2), 221.

Boufidou, F., Nikolaou, C., Alevizos, B., Liappas, I. A., & Christodoulou, G. N. (2004). Cytokine production in bipolar affective disorder patients under lithium treatment. *Journal of Affective Disorders, 82*(2), 309-313.

Bschor, T., Adli, M., Baethge, C., Eichmann, U., Ising, M., Uhr, M., & ... Bauer, M. (2002). Lithium augmentation increases the ACTH and cortisol response in the combined DEX/CRH test in unipolar major depression. *Neuropsychopharmacology, 27*(3), 470-478.

Bschor, T., Baethge, C., Adli, M., Eichmann, U., Ising, M., Uhr, M., & ... Bauer, M. (2003). Association between response to lithium augmentation and the combined DEX/CRH test in major depressive disorder. *Journal of Psychiatric Research, 37*(2), 135-143.

Chenu, F., & Bourin, M. (2006). Potentiation of antidepressant-like activity with lithium: mechanism involved. *Current Drug Targets, 7*(2), 159-163.

Crossley, N. A., & Bauer, M. (2007). Acceleration and augmentation of antidepressants with lithium for depressive disorders: Two meta-analyses of randomized, placebo-controlled trials. *Journal of Clinical Psychiatry, 68*(6), 935-940.

Davis, J.M. (2006). Lithium maintenance of unipolar depression. In: *Lithium in Neuropsychiatry: The Comprehensive Guide*, Bauer, M, Grof, P, Muller-Oerlinghausen, B (eds), Abingdon, UK: Informa UK Ltd, pp.99-108.

Dé Montigny, C., Grunberg, F., Mayer, A., & Deschenes, J. (1981). Lithium Induces Rapid Relief of Depression in Tricyclic Antidepressant Drug Non-Responders. *British Journal of Psychiatry, 138*, 252-256.

Dowlati, Y., Herrmann, N., Swardfager, W., Liu, H., Sham, L., Reim, E. K., & Lanctôt, K. L. (2010). A meta-analysis of cytokines in major depression. *Biological Psychiatry, 67*(5), 446-457.

Fenn, H. H., Robinson, D. p., Luby, V., Dangel, C., Buxton, E., Beattie, M., & ... Yesavage, J. A. (1996). Trends in pharmacotherapy of schizoaffective and bipolar affective disorders: a 5-year naturalistic study. *American Journal of Psychiatry, 153*(5). 711.

Gaynes, B. N., Rush, A. J., Trivedi, M. H., Wisniewski, S. R., Spencer, D., & Fava, M. (2008). The STAR*D study: treating depression in the real world. *Cleveland Clinic Journal of Medicine, 75*(1), 57-66.

Gogtay, N., Ordonez, A., Herman, D. H., Hayashi, K. M., Greenstein, D., Vaituzis, C., & ... Rapoport, J. L. (2007). Dynamic Mapping of Cortical Development before and after the Onset of Pediatric Bipolar Illness. *Journal of Child Psychology and Psychiatry, 48*(9), 852-862.

Gotlib, I. H., & Hamilton, J. P. (2008). Neuroimaging and Depression: Current Status and Unresolved Issues. *Current Directions in Psychological Science, 17*(2), 159.

Jope, R. S., & Roh, M. (2006). Glycogen synthase kinase-3 (GSK3) in psychiatric diseases and therapeutic interventions. *Current Drug Targets, 7*(11), 1421-1434.

Kapusta, N. D., & König, D. (2015). Naturally occurring low-dose lithium in drinking water. *Journal of Clinical Psychiatry, 76*(3), e373-e374.

Hirschfeld, R.M.A. (2005). *Guideline watch: Practice guideline for the treatment of patient with bipolar disorder*. Arlington, VA: American Psychiatric Association. pp. 1-9.

Kempton, M. J., Geddes, J. R., Ettinger, U., Williams, S. C., & Grasby, P. M. (2008). Meta-analysis, database, and meta-regression of 98 structural imaging studies in bipolar disorder. *Archives of General Psychiatry, 65*(9), 1017-32.

Klein, P. S., & Melton, D. A. (1996). A Molecular Mechanism for the Effect of Lithium on Development. *Proceedings of the National Academy of Sciences of the United States of America, 93*(16). 8455-9.

Liu, Y., Ho, R. C., & Mak, A. (2012). Review: Interleukin (IL)-6, tumour necrosis factor alpha (TNF-α) and soluble interleukin-2 receptors (sIL-2R) are elevated in patients with major depressive disorder: A meta-analysis and meta-regression. *Journal of Affective Disorders, 139*(3), 230-239.

Lowe, J. (2015, June 28). 'I Don't Believe in God, but I Believe in Lithium'. *The New York Times Magazine*, pp. 54.

Malhi, G., & Goodwin, G. (2007). The rise and fall of mood stabilizers. *Australian & New Zealand Journal of Psychiatry, 41*(10), 779-783.

Maes, M., Bosmans, E., Suy, E., Vandervorst, C., DeJonckheere, C., & Raus, J. (1991). Depression-related disturbances in mitogen-induced lymphocyte responses and interleukin-1 beta and soluble interleukin-2 receptor production. *Acta Psychiatrica Scandinavica, 84*(4), 379-386.

Mischley, L. (2014). The Role of Lithium in Neurological Health and Disease. *Journal of Orthomolecular Medicine, 29*(3), 101.

McKnight R.F., Adida, M., Budge, K., et al. (2012). Lithium toxicity profile: a systematic review and meta-analysis. *Lancet, 379*(9817), 721-8.

Nahman, S., Belmaker, R. H., & Azab, A. N. (2012). Effects of lithium on lipopolysaccharide-induced inflammation in rat primary glia cells. *Innate Immunity, 18*(3), 447-458.

National Institute of Mental Health & National Institute of Health (NIMH/NIH). (1985). Mood disorders: pharmacologic prevention of recurrences. Consensus Development Panel. *American Journal of Psychiatry, 142*(4), 469-476.

Price, L. H., Charney, D. S., Delgado, P. L., & Heninger, G. R. (1990). Lithium and serotonin function: Implications for the serotonin hypothesis of depression. *Psychopharmacology, 100*(1), 3-12.

Potash, J., Toolan, J., Steele, J., Miller, E., Pearl, J., Zandi, P., & ... McMahon, F. (2007). The bipolar disorder phenome database: a resource for genetic studies. *American Journal of Psychiatry, 164*(8), 1229-1237.

Shorter, E. (2009). The history of lithium therapy. *Bipolar Disorders, 11*(Suppl. 2), 4-9.

Simhandl, C. European Psychiatric Association (EPA) 23rd Congress. Abstract 0181. Presented March 29, 2015.

Schrauzer, G. N., & deVroey, E. (1994). Effects of nutritional lithium supplementation on mood. A placebo-controlled study with former drug users. *Biological Trace Element Research, 40*(1), 89-101.

Severus, E., Taylor, M., Sauer, C., Pfennig, A., Ritter, P., Bauer, M., & Geddes, J. (2014). Lithium for prevention of mood episodes in bipolar disorders: systematic review and meta-analysis. *International Journal of Bipolar Disorders, 2*(1), 1-17.

Smith, L. A., Cornelius, V., Warnock, A., Bell, A., & Young, A. H. (2007). Effectiveness of mood stabilizers and antipsychotics in the maintenance phase of bipolar disorder: A systematic review of randomized controlled trials. *Bipolar Disorders, 9*(4), 394-412.

Souza, F., & Goodwin, G. (1991). Lithium treatment and prophylaxis in unipolar depression: a meta-analysis. *British Journal of Psychiatry, 158,* 666-75.

Sugawara, H., Sakamoto, K., Harada, T., & Ishigooka, J. (2010). Predictors of efficacy in lithium augmentation for treatment-resistant depression. *Journal of Affective Disorders, 125*(1-3), 165-8.

Thase, M. E., & Sachs, G. S. (2000). Therapeutic approach: Bipolar depression: pharmacotherapy and related therapeutic strategies. *Biological Psychiatry, 48*(6), 558-572.

World Health Organization (WHO). (2015). *Depression fact sheet.* Retrieved from www.who.int/mediacentre/factsheets/fs369/en

Young, A. H., & Hammond, J. M. (2007). Lithium in mood disorders: Increasing evidence base, declining use? *British Journal of Psychiatry, 191*(6), 474-476.

# Ten

## LITHIUM AS A MEDICINE: SUICIDE PREVENTION

Suicide is a serious public health problem around the world. It causes immeasurable loss not only to the individuals whose lives are abruptly cut short but also to their families and communities. When people die by suicide, their family and friends often experience shock, anger, guilt, and intractable depression.

The World Health Organization (WHO) estimates that each year approximately one million people die from suicide, which represents a global mortality rate of 16 people per 100,000, or one death every 40 seconds. By 2020, the rate of suicide is predicted to increase to one death every 20 seconds. Worldwide, suicide is among the top five causes of mortality in teenagers between 15 and 19, and in many countries it ranks first or second as a cause of death among both boys and girls in this age group. Closer to home, suicide is the tenth leading cause of death, claiming more than twice as many American lives each year as homicide. On average, between 2001 and 2009, more than 33,000 Americans died each year as a result of suicide, or more than one person every 15 minutes.

More than eight million adults report having serious thoughts of suicide in the past year, while 2.5 million report making a suicide plan in the past year, and 1.1 million report a suicide attempt in the past year. Women are more likely to express suicidal thoughts and to make nonfatal attempts than men. The prevalence of suicidal thoughts, suicide planning, and suicide attempts is significantly higher among young adults aged 18-29 than among adults over 30. Almost 16% of students in grades 9 to 12 report having seriously considered suicide, and 7.8 % report having attempted to kill themselves at least once during the previous 12 months. People who attempt suicide and survive may suffer from serious injuries, such as broken bones, brain damage, or organ failure. Among young adults ages 15 to 24, there are approximately 100-200 attempts for every completed suicide. Nonfatal, self-inflicted injuries result in an estimated $6.5 billion in combined medical and work loss costs.

About 90% of those who successfully complete suicide have a clinically diagnosable psychiatric disorder. In fact, the rate of suicide among persons with mood disorders has been estimated to be 30 times higher than in the general population (WHO, 2014). Because of this alarming statistic, reducing suicide risk is an urgent priority in the treatment for patients with mood disorders.

## Neglected Area of Research

Treating patients with suicidal behavior remains as one of the most challenging obstacles for health care professionals. Despite its enormous societal impact, little progress has been made in the scientific understanding or treatment of suicidal behavior in the last several decades. Large epidemiologic studies have shown mental disorders to be major risk factors, but psychiatry has long neglected the topic. Other than as symptoms of Borderline Personality Disorder and mood disorders, suicide and suicide attempts were not listed in the *Diagnostic and Statistical Manual of Mental Disorders, IV (DSM-IV)*. The *DSM-V* does not code suicidal behavior, even though it is the most common emergency in psychiatry. For every study on suicide-related behavior published in the *American Journal of Psychiatry* and *JAMA Psychiatry* in the past 5 years, there were six papers on schizophrenia, which is only one-quarter as common as suicidal behavior. And in contrast to studies on schizophrenia, those on suicidal behavior are mostly epidemiological and do not investigate mechanisms that underlie the behavior (Aleman & Denys, 2014).

# Lithium as a Medicine: Suicide Prevention

Research has long been available that points to nutritional biomarkers as predictors of suicide risk. Low cholesterol and low omega fatty acids have been implicated as risk factors for several decades, but clear-cut results in small studies have not until recently been followed up by controlled clinical trials.

Patients with Anorexia Nervosa (AN) have the highest risk for suicide among patients with psychiatric illnesses. Moreover, the most frequent cause of death among AN patients is suicide (37%). The suicide rate is eight times higher among young women with AN than in young women in general. Despite the high suicide risk, there have been no advances in the biological treatment of AN in 50 years.

In 1994, the *Morbidity and Mortality Weekly Report,* published by the Centers for Disease Control and Prevention (CDC), identified the lack of evaluation research as the single greatest obstacle to improving current efforts to prevent suicide. Sadly, this remains true two decades later. Right now the tools are available to identify patients at risk of suicide, and science shows that correcting nutritional and metabolic imbalances can have a positive influence on mood.

Several studies have explored the anti-suicidal effects of lithium. One of the first descriptions of lithium's anti-suicidal properties was reported when researchers found that suicide attempts decreased by 20% during treatment with lithium when compared to treatment without lithium therapy (Hanus & Zapletalek, 1984). Other studies arrived at similar conclusions, hypothesizing that lithium is an effective agent to reduce the risk of suicide due to its ability to stabilize mood and reduce aggression and impulsivity (Comai et al., 2012). Because of lithium's unique profile, literature suggests that lithium is a safe and effective prevention strategy to combat suicidal behavior.

## Diminishing Suicidal Behavior with Lithium

An impressive array of research over the past several decades has proven conclusively that treatment with lithium can reduce the high risk of suicide in patients with mood disorders and reduce suicide risk in the general population. This evidence base, drawn from several studies, has clearly established lithium's effectiveness in preventing both attempted and completed suicides. No other drug demonstrates such clear-cut positive results. Sadly, this effective treatment is still largely unrecognized and therefore under-prescribed among many physicians who treat patients with mood disorders.

Yet the promise lithium delivers is undeniable. Following John Cade's discovery in 1949 that lithium could diminish the severity of manic episodes, researchers first studied lithium's potential effectiveness in reducing suicide risk in patients with bipolar disorder. Research studies conducted over the last 40 years have shown consistently that lithium lowers suicide risk in bipolar patients. One study, for example, examined life-threatening or fatal suicidal acts in more than 300 bipolar patients, before, during, and after long-term lithium treatment. The patients had been ill for more than eight years. While these patients were taking lithium, their rate of suicides and suicide attempts decreased nearly 7-fold. The first year the patients were off lithium, the suicide rate rose to 20 times the rate during maintenance lithium. The risk doubled with abrupt, rapid withdrawal from lithium compared to a gradual discontinuation. Later the rate returned to the level found before lithium treatment began (Tondo & Baldessarini, 2014). Epidemiological research reflects these findings, showing a connection between regions with higher lithium prescription rates and reduced suicide risk.

Through the years, many relatively small studies have confirmed that lithium decreases suicide attempts and completions in patients with bipolar disorder. More recently, meta-analyses provide impressive proof of the benefits of lithium for suicide prevention in these bipolar patients. In a meta-analysis of 22 studies in patients with major affective disorders, covering 33,473 patient-years of risk, researchers found that suicide was 82% less frequent during lithium treatment (Tondo et al., 2001). Not only is it more effective than placebo, but maintenance treatment with lithium also lowers suicide risk in bipolar patients more than anticonvulsant and antipsychotic drugs.

In another meta-analysis, which focused on 31 studies of lithium treatment in patients with bipolar disorder, the risks of completed and attempted suicide were consistently lower, by approximately 80%, during treatment that extended for an average of 18 months (Baldessarini et al., 2006). These decisive benefits of lithium treatment have been seen in both randomized and open clinical trials.

Lithium's capacity to lower suicide risk in bipolar patients has also been studied in specific subgroups. One study assessed more than 1,300 veterans from five different veterans' hospitals. Compared to patients on placebo as well as those on atypical antipsychotics and sedatives, the patients on lithium had the lowest percentage of suicide attempts and other deliberate self-harm (Ahern et al., 2013).

Lithium's protective effects against suicide were compared with protective effects of several mood-stabilizing anticonvulsants, including valproate, carbamazepine, and lamotrigine. In more than 30,000 patients, lithium consistently showed superior suicide prevention effects. An analysis of randomized trials yielded nearly a three-fold superiority favoring lithium over anticonvulsants. Researchers, then, have observed major reductions in suicide risk when lithium is used not just for treating or preventing acute manic episodes, but also for long-term maintenance therapy in patients with unipolar, bipolar II, and bipolar I disorders (Tondo, & Baldessarini, 2014).

Bipolar patients on lithium seem to have lower risk of death from all causes than patients taking placebo, tricyclic antidepressants, carbamazepine, and lamotrigine. A meta-analysis of 48 randomized controlled trials found patients on maintenance lithium not only had fewer suicides and suicide attempts, but 60% fewer deaths of any causes than patients on these other drugs. Based on these frequently repeated study results, researchers concluded that lithium is the treatment with the most significant evidence base, and it should be first-line treatment for mood-disordered patients at risk of suicide (Cipriani et al., 2013).

Because lithium decreases the intensity of both manic and depressive cycles in bipolar disorder, researchers considered the possible benefits of lithium treatment for reducing suicide risk in patients with major depressive disorder. The first meta-analysis on the subject, published in 2007, revealed that the anti-suicidal effects of lithium in patients with recurrent major depressive disorder are of similar magnitude to the effects in bipolar patients – a 76% reduction of risk of suicides and attempts was found. (Guzzetta et al., 2007).

Lithium's effectiveness in preventing suicide in depressed patients is particularly important in light of concerns about whether antidepressant drugs curtail suicidal behavior. Although SSRIs have been shown to be the most effective monotherapy for treating depression, evidence that they help prevent suicide is inconclusive. Particular symptoms like agitation, restlessness, irritability, anger, insomnia, and dysphoria are especially common in patients with mood disorders and are sometimes exacerbated with antidepressant treatment (Tondo & Baldessarini, 2014).

## Mechanisms

The mechanisms underlying lithium's anti-suicidal effects are challenging to study as they are obviously impossible to reproduce in animal models. Despite this limitation, researchers have been able to explore the specific anti-suicidal effects of lithium in various ways. Some researchers speculate that lithium prevents relapse of mood disorders. Lithium decreases both aggression and impulsivity (Cipriani et al., 2013). The strongest measured association between suicide and personality appears to be with indicators of aggression and impulsivity. Recent research in genetics defines aggression and impulsivity as suicide endophenotypes. An endophenotype is a measurable trait marker that bridges the disease of interest (in this case suicide) and the genotype. Lithium dampens expression of these traits, thereby reducing the suicide rate in genetically vulnerable patients with mood disorders (Kovacsics, Gottesman, & Gould, 2009). Examining the mechanisms that contribute to lithium's anti-aggressive and anti-impulsive effects is beginning to clarify the neurobiological underpinnings of suicidal behavior. We know that neurobiological abnormalities heighten the likelihood of suicide.

In the prefrontal cortex of suicide completers, the number of serotonin transporter binding sites has been reported to be lower than in controls (Kovacsics et al., 2009). The strong biological and genetic predisposition for suicide risk is likely related to abnormalities in the central serotonin 5-HT system. Low levels of serotonin contribute to both aggression and impulsivity. Lithium may modify aggression through its actions on the serotonin system.

Lithium leads to an increase in serotonin and exerts complex effects on the serotonin system at multiple levels. Researchers speculate that lithium may increase 5-HT turnover in the brain in areas that regulate emotional stimuli, cognitive function, and impulse control - systems directly linked to suicidal behaviors (Lauterbach et al., 2008).

New research suggests that lithium may reduce brain inflammation by adjusting the metabolism of the omega-3 fatty acid DHA. Lithium helps to moderate inflammation by dampening cytokine reactivity as well. Inflammation is consistently associated with an increased risk of suicide. The impulse that leads individuals to contemplate suicide may activate a biological stress response, which includes an inflammatory response. Thus, patients with suicidal depression may have higher levels of inflammation than non-suicidal depressed patients.

## Prescription Rate

Better identifying the mechanisms by which lithium reduces suicide risk will lead to a clear picture of the neurobiology of suicide. More precise understanding of how lithium acts on neurotransmission and cell signaling pathways will lead to better suicide prevention and treatment strategies. While scientists proceed with this research, practitioners should act on the unequivocal knowledge already available by prescribing maintenance lithium for patients with mood disorders who may be at risk of suicide. It is the only drug that has demonstrated such clear benefits. With safe and inexpensive lithium maintenance treatment, the suicide risk for patients with mood disorders is reduced to the suicide rate in the general population.

The underutilization of lithium is not just an American problem. Lithium prophylaxis prevents about 250 suicides per year in Germany, although lithium is prescribed within the National Health Scheme at low levels. About 820,000 patients in Germany are in need of prophylactic lithium treatment, according to researchers who study patterns of prescription and disease. Yet only about 50,000 patients in Germany received lithium medication in 2001. Some German medical doctors have called this discrepancy irritating and questioned whether this constitutes malpractice (Müller-Oerlinghausen,

Berghöfer, & Ahrens, 2003). Epidemiological studies reflect research findings that lithium lowers suicide risk. Analysis reveals a connection between regions with higher lithium prescription rates and reduced suicide risk.

## Tap Water

Ecologic studies demonstrate that lithium consumption lowers the rate of suicide in the general population. The association between lithium levels in tap water and the rate of suicide has been studied in at least four countries and three continents. Lithium levels in tap water were examined in 27 Texas counties and results showed incidence rates of suicide are significantly higher in counties whose drinking water supplies contain little or no lithium than in counties with water lithium levels of at least 70 micrograms/L (Schrauzer & Shrestha, 1990). A second, larger study of lithium in the public water supply in Texas found not only a negative association between lithium and suicide rates, but a negative association with hospital admissions and readmissions for psychoses, neuroses, and personal disorders as well as homicide rates and crime rates (Blüml et al. 2013).

Correlations between lithium levels in tap water and suicide were also seen in 18 municipalities in Japan, and in Austria in a nationwide sample of 6,460 households (Ohgami et al., 2009; Kapusta et al., 2011). All the studies demonstrated that the overall suicide rate and the suicide mortality ratio were inversely associated with lithium tap water levels. Lithium not only prevents suicide in those with mood disorders, but in the general population as well, even at low levels.

## A Problem with Several Risk Factors

A predisposition for suicide is usually attributed to a convergence between stressful or traumatic life events and neurobiological factors. According to data presented from the World Mental Health (WMH) Surveys, risk factors for suicidal behavior include sex, age, education and income level, marital status, unemployment, presence of comorbid psychiatric disorders, and childhood adversities (Borges et al., 2010).

## Lithium as a Medicine: Suicide Prevention

Genetics is also a factor that influences suicide risk. Geneticists have often focused on altered serotonergic activity in the prefrontal cortex as a precursor of suicide risk. That genetics underlies a predisposition for suicide is confirmed by studies of monozygotic twins. A monozygotic twin of a person who attempted suicide has a 17-fold greater risk than a dizygotic twin of also making a suicide attempt. Some investigators estimate that heritability of suicide risk is as high as 55% (Akbarian & Halene, 2013).

Although genetics clearly has an influence on suicide risk, a particular gene or genetic variant associated with this risk has not been identified. Studies of 9,000 people with mood disorders who attempted suicide ruled out a common genetic variation (Perlis et al., 2010).

More recently, investigators have found consistent gene expression changes in the brains of people who committed suicide. In a study of hippocampal tissue from brains of 62 men (46 who committed suicide and 16 controls), they discovered extensive methylation in DNA neurons. Promoter DNA methylation levels were significantly greater for several genes in the brains of those who had committed suicide (LaBonte et al., 2013).

DNA methylation, a major regulator of genetic expression, occurs for different reasons; it can result from stressful or traumatic life experiences. DNA methylation provides a molecular link between genes and life experience. This finding of a link between the neuronal genome and life experience contributes to researchers' understanding that suicidal behavior results from an interplay between genetics and the environment. The evidence of broad reprogramming of promoter DNA methylation in the hippocampus tissues of completed suicides helps prove that gene expression alterations lead to increased suicide risk.

Both suicide and depression are associated with extensive changes in the molecular structure of nerve cells, yet the hippocampus tissue of suicidal patients is distinct from those who are vulnerable to depression (Yen et al., 2009). This distinction sheds light on particular neurobiological mechanisms that lead to suicide. It further shows that genome exploration in brain tissue can be especially illuminating when focused on particular cells in order to identify specific epigenetic signals related to a disease or outcome.

These recent studies have helped better isolate the epigenetic risk structure that establishes a predisposition to suicide. Most epigenetic markers are now understood to undergo changes that are both dynamic and reversible. These changes can range between an enduring trait triggered by an early life situation and dysregulation in response to an acute recent event. Because epigenetic dysregulation may be reversed, new medications targeting the chromatin-associated proteins may help undo genetic dysregulation caused by methylation (Akbarian & Halene, 2013).

Suicide is a complex behavior that results from multiple pathological pathways. A review of literature has found that there are several theories that explain suicide risk, including social, environmental, genetic, and neurobiological factors (Mandelli et al., 2015). However, much of the literature suggests that suicidal behavior is likely to be attributed to the interaction between genetic predisposition and exposure to environmental risk factors.

Genetic liability is modulated by multiple environmental factors, which can result in the development of abnormal temperamental traits associated with suicidal behavior. Epigenetic alterations also increase vulnerability by interfering with normal gene expression. The neurobiological abnormalities that ensue are associated with developing specific emotional and behavioral phenotypes and cognitive impairments. Understanding the effects of methylation changes in genes involved in regulating behavior and cognitive processes is vital to understanding suicide risk. This understanding may lead to identifying ways to reverse the epigenetic process that heightens risk of suicide as an outcome. Because these risk factors also influence brain processes, understanding these changes in neurobiology is of urgent importance in preventing suicide.

## The Challenges

Suicide is a complex problem. But no problem is more costly in terms of unnecessary suffering and loss of years of potential life. On an individual level, suicide devastates families; on a national level, it is an issue of great public health importance.

# Lithium as a Medicine: Suicide Prevention

As suicide involves the interplay of so many factors, it challenges efforts to develop effective prevention strategies. But the underlying neurobiology cannot be ignored. Accumulating evidence continues to establish the correlation between nutritional deficiencies and their impact on mental health. As a result, the development of psychiatric disorders increases the risk of suicidal behavior. The findings from epidemiological studies demonstrate conclusively that the overall suicide rate and the suicide mortality ratio are inversely associated with lithium levels. Because lithium even at low doses has beneficial effects, lithium supplementation or lithiation of drinking water should be explored as a possible means of suicide prevention.

As emphasized by the Surgeon General's report, we need more research in neurobiology and epigenetics to gain a better understanding of mechanisms that lead to suicide. As clinicians, we need to do a better job of monitoring patients, especially those with depression, bipolar disorder, anorexia nervosa, and comorbid substance abuse. We need to address nutritional deficiencies and inflammation. Primary care physicians as well need to be vigilant in monitoring patients for whom they have prescribed medications that may heighten risk of suicide-related behaviors. There is no more important task for us as a society than integrating the interventions we know are effective in order to prevent suicide. Lithium as a nutritional or pharmaceutical intervention for the prevention of suicide has to be a public health priority and mental health treatment for all high risk individuals.

## CHAPTER 10 | References

Ahearn, E., Chen, P., Hertzberg, M., et al. (2013). Suicide attempts in veterans with bipolar disorder during treatment with lithium, divalproex, and atypical antipsychotics. *Journal of Affective Disorders, 145*(1), 77-82.

Akbarian, S., & Halene, T. (2013). The Neuroepigenetics of Suicide. *American Journal of Psychiatry, 170*(5), 462–465.

Aleman, A., & Denys, D. (2014). A road map for suicide research and prevention. *Nature, 509*(7501), 421-423.

Baldessarini, R. J., Tondo, L., Davis, P., Pompili, M., Goodwin, F. K., & Hennen, J. (2006). Decreased risk of suicides and attempts during long-term lithium treatment: a meta-analytic review. *Bipolar Disorders, 8*(5 Pt 2), 625-39.

Borges, G., Nock, M. K., Haro Abad, J. M., Hwang, I., Sampson, N. A., Alonso, J., & ... Kessler, R. C. (2010). Twelve-month prevalence of and risk factors for suicide attempts in the World Health Organization World Mental Health Surveys. *Journal of Clinical Psychiatry, 71*(12), 1617-1628.

Blüml, V., Regier, M. D., Hlavin, G., Rockett, I. R., König, F., Vyssoki, B., & ... Kapusta, N. D. (2013). Lithium in the public water supply and suicide mortality in Texas. *Journal of Psychiatric Research, 47*(3), 407-411.

Cipriani, A., Hawton, K., Stockton, S., & Geddes, J. R. (2013). Lithium in the prevention of suicide in mood disorders: Updated systematic review and meta-analysis. *BMJ: British Medical Journal, 346*, 1-13.

Comai, S., Tau, M., Pavlovic, Z., & Gobbi, G. (2012). The psychopharmacology of aggressive behavior: a translational approach: part 2: clinical studies using atypical antipsychotics, anticonvulsants, and lithium. *Journal of Clinical Psychopharmacology, 32*(2), 237-260.

Guzzetta, F., Tondo, L., Centorrino, F., & Baldessarini, R. J. (2007). Lithium treatment reduces suicide risk in recurrent major depressive disorder. *Journal of Clinical Psychiatry, 68*(3), 380-383.

Hanus, K., & Zapletálek, M. (1984). [Suicidal activity of patients with affective disorders during the preventive use of lithium]. *Ceskoslovenská Psychiatrie, 80*(2), 97-100.

U.S. Department of Health and Human Services (HHS). (2012, September). *2012 National Strategy for Suicide Prevention: Goals and Objectives for Action.* Office of the Surgeon General and National Action Alliance for Suicide Prevention. Washington, DC: HHS.

Kapusta, N. D., Mossaheb, N., Etzersdorfer, E., Hlavin, G., Thau, K., Willeit, M., & ... Leithner-Dziubas, K. (2011). Lithium in drinking water and suicide mortality. *British Journal of Psychiatry, 198*(5), 346-350.

Kovacsics, C. E., Gottesman, I. I., & Gould, T. D. (2009). Lithium's antisuicidal efficacy: elucidation of neurobiological targets using endophenotype strategies. *Annual Review of Pharmacology and Toxicology, 49,* 175-198.

Labonte, B., Suderman, M., Maussion, G., Lopez, J. P., Navarro-Sánchez, L., Yerko, V., & ... Turecki, G. (2013). Genome-wide methylation changes in the brains of suicide completers. *American Journal of Psychiatry, 170*(5), 511-520.

Lauterbach, E., Felber, W., Müller-Oerlinghausen, B., Ahrens, B., Bronisch, T., Meyer, T., & ... Hohagen, F. (2008). Adjunctive lithium treatment in the prevention of suicidal behaviour in depressive disorders: A randomised, placebo-controlled, 1-year trial. *Acta Psychiatrica Scandinavica, 118*(6), 469-479.

Mandelli, L., Carli, V., Serretti, A., & Sarchiapone, M. (2011). Suicidal behavior: genes, environmental stress and temperamental traits. *Suicidologi, 16*(2), 18-26.

Müller-Oerlinghausen, B., Berghöfer, A., & Ahrens, B. (2003). The antisuicidal and mortality-reducing effect of lithium prophylaxis: Consequences for guidelines in clinical psychiatry. *Canadian Journal of Psychiatry, 48*(7), 433-439.

Ohgami, H., Terao, T., Shiotsuki, I., Ishii, N., & Iwata, N. (2009). Lithium levels in drinking water and risk of suicide. *British Journal of Psychiatry, 194*(5), 464-5.

Perils, R. H., Huang, J., Purcell, S., Fava, M., Rush, A. J., Sullivan, P. F., & ... Smoller, J. W. (2010). Genome-wide association study of suicide attempts in mood disorder patients. *American Journal of Psychiatry, 167*(12), 1499.

Pompili, M., Mancinelli, I., Girardi, P., Ruberto, A., & Tatarelli, R. (2004). Suicide in anorexia nervosa: A meta-analysis. *International Journal of Eating Disorders, 36*(1), 99-103.

Schrauzer, G.N. & Shrestha, K.P. (1990). Lithium in drinking water and the incidences of crimes, suicides, and arrests related to drug addictions. *Biological Trace Elements Research, 25*(2), 105-13.

Tondo, L., Hennen, J., & Baldessarini, R. J. (2001). Lower suicide risk with long-term lithium treatment in major affective illness: A meta-analysis. *Acta Psychiatrica Scandinavica, 104*(3), 163-172.

Tondo, L., & Baldessarini, R. J. (2014). Reduction of suicidal behavior in bipolar disorder patients during long-term treatment with lithium. In S. H. Koslow, P. Ruiz, C. B. Nemeroff, S. H. Koslow, P. Ruiz, C. B. Nemeroff (Eds.), *A concise guide to understanding suicide: Epidemiology, pathophysiology, and prevention.* New York, NY, US: Cambridge University Press. pp. 217-228.

# Eleven

## LITHIUM AS A MEDICINE: IRRITABILITY, ANGER AND AGGRESSION

In behavioral science, aggression is a term used to describe a range of behaviors that result in physical and emotional harm to oneself, others, or objects in the environment. Aggressive behaviors take many forms and include lashing out in physical, verbal, and emotional ways. People exhibiting aggressive tendencies are often restless, irritable, and impulsive, and cause a great deal of damage to themselves and others.

In reality, aggression is far more damaging and pervasive than these simple clinical definitions can describe. Aggressive behavior is a major public health concern due to the destructive and traumatic impact it has on individuals, families, and communities. Domestic violence, criminal activity, and self-harming addictions can all be linked back to aggression. What's more, aggressive impulses are frequently seen in combination with other mental health disorders including depression, suicidal behavior, and substance abuse. Regardless of the primary psychiatric condition, chronic aggression is prognostic of longer and more exhaustive treatments, as well as poorer outcomes (Pappadopulos et al., 2006).

It is a common misconception that aggressive tendencies are the inevitable result of genetic proneness, negative life experiences, or a violent upbringing. This is simply not accurate. An expanding body of neurological research is showing that aggression is not purely environmental or psychosocial in its origins, but rather the result of a complex blend of biological factors. Neurotransmitter balance, nutrient metabolism, and brain structure all seem to play a significant role.

The recognition that aggressive behavior has biochemical underpinnings has opened up a new window of understanding about the condition and allowed researchers and clinicians to look at it in a more physiological context. It has offered new hope for treatment strategies as well; perhaps by correcting disturbances in the nervous system, dysfunctional behaviors could be turned around. If taken further, maybe there could even be preventative strategies to help those with a predisposition to or family history of aggression, to help counteract outbursts before they occur. Imagine the implications: the pain, harm, and hardships that could be avoided.

Lithium, the reliable mood stabilizer, has proven to be one of the most effective therapies in treating aggression and irritability. For over forty years researchers have explored its uses in reducing violent behaviors in criminal populations with relative success. However, the extremely high doses used in most studies have resulted in negative side effects that made treatment consistency difficult. With no side effects and remarkable therapeutic potential, low dose lithium may provide the support for individuals struggling with aggressive behavior.

## Lithium Treats Aggression

It has long been recognized that lithium shifts abusive and destructive patterns in patients with mental health disorders. Cade's initial trials using lithium carbonate to treat bipolar patients in 1949 demonstrated this shift. Manic patients, who had previously been considered "dangerous" and "violent" towards themselves or others, were able to leave hospital confinement and returned safely to their homes with the help of ongoing lithium treatment.

Since the time of lithium's approval by the FDA in 1970, the anti-aggressive effects of pharmaceutical lithium have been studied in various settings among diverse populations. Over twenty studies have tested the use of high-dose lithium as an agent to quell aggressive and impulsive behavior across various demographics (Prado-Lima et al., 2001). Patient groups in whom the anti-aggressive effects of lithium have been most dramatic include prisoners with uncontrolled rage outbursts, adolescents with conduct disorders, mentally handicapped individuals, patients with traumatic brain injury, and those with substance abuse problems. The volume and efficacy of lithium studies amidst these hard-to-treat groups have been significant, especially given the limited number of interventions that have been found to be of any benefit at all.

## *LITHIUM SHOWS PROMISE IN PRISON POPULATIONS*

The United States incarcerates more people than any other nation, and the system of jails and prisons that holds these individuals has become the largest provider of mental health care in the country. In these institutions rates of aggression are many times higher than those seen in the community (Ford, 2015). Studies focusing on the use of lithium administration among prisoners are thus particularly telling when it comes to examining its effects on aggressive behavior.

Three long-term studies have tested the efficacy of lithium therapy in violent and aggressive criminals. The first in this line of studies was conducted in 1972 among 27 male inmates of a California medical facility who had serious repeated violent behavior (Tupin et al., 1972). Patients were treated with lithium carbonate for one to one and a half years at a starting dose of 1800 mg/day. After treatment, the men reported that they experienced an increased capacity to reflect on the consequences of their actions, control angry feelings, and experience diminished intensity of angry emotions. Decreased frequency of disciplinary actions for violent behaviors was observed among 68% of the lithium-treated patients. Furthermore, 42.5% experienced decreased frequency of disciplinary actions for *nonviolent* behavior as well. Two follow-up studies using a similar study design also concluded that individuals treated with lithium experienced significantly fewer infractions of both violent and nonviolent types compared to control groups (Sheard, 1975; Sheard et al., 1976).

The aggression-mediating properties of lithium have also been observed in females. One open-label trial observed eight child-abusing mothers who voluntarily attended the "Program for Treatment of Abused Children and their Parents." The mothers received lithium for the 60 day duration of the trial. At the study's conclusion, analyses showed that mothers experienced reduced abusive behaviors and lowered physical aggression towards other people and objects with lithium therapy (Prado-Lima, 2001).

### *Lithium Helps with Childhood Behavioral Disorders*

Aggression is also a serious problem in children and adolescents. A recent investigation by the Centers for Disease Control reported that disruptive behavior disorders, including oppositional defiant disorder and conduct disorder, are the second most common mental health problem among children aged 6 to 17, with rates falling only marginally behind those for attention-deficit/hyperactivity disorder (ADHD) (Perou, 2013). Disruptive behavior disorders are characterized by a persistent pattern of impulsive, hostile, and aggressive action.

Over time it has become generally accepted that symptoms of aggression in childhood predict a poor outcome and antisocial behavior later in life. However newer evidence is proving that this doesn't necessarily have to be the case. Although psychotherapeutic and family-based interventions have traditionally been considered first-line treatments for behavior disorders, the scientific literature has shown that adjunctive treatment with lithium can substantially reduce behaviors (Masi et al., 2009).

The results of three double blind studies, one open clinical trial, and one retrospective study have all indicated that four or more weeks of treatment with lithium lessens aggression in children and adolescents with conduct disorder (Campbell et al., 1984, 1995; Malone et al., 1994, 2000; Masi et al., 2009). Lithium's capacity to reduce impulsive aggression was seen on clinical observation and was statistically significant across these studies, which took place over a span of 25 years.

One additional study sought to determine the safety of lithium for children and adolescents, especially when required for the long term (Delong & Aldershof, 1987). The study included 196 subjects with a variety of psychiatric diagnoses who were treated for periods of up to ten years. The authors concluded that lithium was in fact a safe and effective therapy for a variety of mental health conditions in children.

# Lithium as a Medicine: Irritability, Anger and Aggression

## Defining Irritability

If violence and conduct issues fall on one end of the spectrum of aggressive behavior, irritability sits at the other. Irritability can be loosely defined as a state of hypersensitivity and reactivity, resulting in excessive and easily provoked anger, annoyance, or impatience.

Irritability is viewed as a milder form of aggression, which can occur in a chronic or episodic way. It is the most common reason for children to be brought in for psychiatric evaluation, and is linked to significant impairment in adulthood as well (Peterson, 1996; Roberson-Nay et al., 2015). Individuals with irritability often struggle with academic problems, poverty, psychopathology, and suicidality. There is also a strong overlap between irritability and other mental health conditions, including addiction, bipolar disorder, and autism spectrum disorders (Leibenluft et al. 2006, Stringaris et al. 2009).

In spite of its commonality and pervasiveness, irritability has received relatively little formal attention from researchers and practitioners. Part of the problem is that irritability is a low-frequency behavior that can be difficult to assess. There is no reliable marker, measure, or test to diagnose irritability; there isn't even a set of established diagnostic criteria to define irritability as a distinctive psychological trait (Snaith & Taylor, 1985). As Daniel P. Dickstein, MD wrote in a recent review on the subject, in psychiatry "irritability is everywhere and nowhere at once" (Dickstein, 2015).

Those living or working closely with affected individuals know very well that irritability causes considerable distress to patients, peers, and others trying to treat or help them. Finding out more about the biological underpinnings of irritable mood would therefore be a huge step toward helping those with a number of different mental health conditions—from road rage, to substance abuse and beyond.

New research is just starting to skim the surface of understanding irritability as a unique neurobiological trait. In one study published in the *American Journal of Psychiatry*, investigators pooled data from 1,310 twin pairs who were followed between the ages of 8-20. Researchers found that genetic effects on irritability were developmentally dynamic from middle childhood through young adulthood. In other words, there didn't appear to be a single set of genetic risk factors that emerged early and persisted throughout development. Rather, genes appeared to be turned on and off over the course of development to drive or deter irritable behavior. Furthermore, unique environmental influences, especially events occurring during childhood, also had a lasting effect on the expression of irritability (Roberson-Nay et al., 2015). These findings suggest that there are biologically determined trajectories of irritability, which could advance classification and diagnosis.

In my practice low dose lithium has proven to be a highly efficacious therapy for those with irritability. More study is needed to determine why this is the case, but it does stand to reason that lithium, with its ability to quell aggression and stabilize mood, would prove helpful for managing irritability as well. Lithium also has known epigenetic pathways, which could help stabilize the expression of irritability over the long term. Further research should investigate the role of lithium in the biology of irritability, and consider if lithium deficiency could be a contributing cause.

## Concerns with Toxicity

While studies testing lithium's anti-aggressive effects across varying diagnoses have been promising, toxicity has remained a relevant concern. In many cases, studies testing lithium as a medium to control violent outbursts or impulsive behaviors have pushed dosages to the very upper limit of what is considered to be "therapeutic."

Adverse effects most commonly reported with taking lithium for aggressive behaviors and/or irritable mood have included gastrointestinal complaints (such as nausea, stomachache, vomiting), polydipsia and increased urinary frequency, tremor and moderate weight gain (Masi et al., 2009). Lithium toxicity, in the form of renal dysfunction or hypothyroidism, has been rare but has occurred in some cases. Across the literature, authors have consistently emphasized that dosage and serum levels must be carefully monitored and tailored to each individual in order to avoid acute symptoms while maintaining remission of aggressive and irritable behaviors.

However, what many have failed to realize is that a "more is better" dogma does not necessarily fit with these patient groups. Doses do not need to be pushed to the limit to be effective. On the contrary, pharmaceutical lithium can increase agitation in some cases and can lead to treatment discontinuation. There is another way.

## Tap Water Studies: Is Low Dose Lithium the Answer?

A series of interesting studies investigating naturally occurring lithium levels in drinking water have established that low doses of lithium may have significance for the treatment and prevention of aggression and irritability. Natural lithium contents in tap water can be as high as 1 mg or more of dissolved lithium per liter, depending on the geographic origin of the drinking water (Kapusta, 2015).

We've reviewed these studies elsewhere in this book, but find it important to consider them again here within the context of aggression. In the first study in 1970, levels of organically derived lithium in the water of 27 Texan counties were analyzed and compared to the incidence of admissions and readmissions for psychoses, neuroses and personality disorders at local state mental hospitals. Data from a two-year period were collected and analyzed (Dawson, 1970). The authors noticed a marked trend: the higher the lithium content in the water supply, the lower the rate of psychiatric illness in that county. This association remained significant even after correcting for possible confounding variables such as population density and distance to the nearest state hospitals.

A follow-up study in the same Texan counties looked at similar variables over a longer 9 year span (Schrauzer & Shrestha, 1990). Researchers came up with similar results: the incidence of suicide, homicide, and rape was significantly higher in counties where drinking water contained little or no lithium, versus those with levels ranging from 70-170 mcg/L.

Unsure if these striking findings were somehow unique to that geographical region, other researchers have sought to replicate the study template in other areas throughout the globe. Lithium water studies have now been repeated internationally at sites in Austria, England, Greece and Japan. Overall the collection has revealed a strong inverse correlation between aggressive crime and suicide, on the one hand; and supplemental levels of lithium in the water supply on the other (Kapusta et al., 2011; Kabacs et al., 2011; Giotakos et al., 2015; Sugawara et al., 2013).

Another interesting finding came from a study that looked at lithium levels in the hair of criminals. Hair analysis is one of the most accurate methods for testing long-term mineral status and is therefore highly advantageous for determining where deficiencies are present. This study found that violent criminals had little to no stores of lithium as revealed through hair mineral analysis, suggesting the idea that perhaps lithium *deficiency* was contributing to defiant behaviors (Schrauzer et al., 1992). With this background, researchers have designed clinical trials using low-dose lithium as an intervention for those struggling with behavioral disorders. In one such study, 24 participants with histories of aggression, impulsivity, and social transgressions were recruited (Schrauzer & de Vroey, 1994). A daily dose of 400 mcg of lithium was administered over the course of four weeks. Improvement on indices of happiness, friendliness, energy levels, and other mood-related parameters was observed.

Additional trials are required to fully understand the therapeutic potential of low-dose lithium; however, the research appears to indicate that lithium deficiency may contribute to volatile mood and aggressive behavior. This explanation is a major departure from current philosophies that consider aggression as a psychosocial issue to be treated with incarceration and pharmaceutics. The lithium deficiency hypothesis explains why studies testing pharmaceutical lithium have been successful. A lower dose of lithium has tremendous benefits without the side effects. A rationale therefore exists for lithium supplementation in persons exhibiting irritable or aggressive behaviors. This is especially true if the individuals are living in geographical areas known to be lithium-deficient.

## Mechanisms

Although we don't tend to think about lithium as an essential nutrient, a look at human neurobiology suggests that the nervous system was actually designed to have this mineral present. This becomes particularly obvious when considering some of the key mechanisms involved in regulating aggressive behavior.

# Lithium as a Medicine: Irritability, Anger and Aggression

### *Lithium Facilitates Vitamin B12 and Folate Transport*
The B vitamins, including B12 and folate, help to build and maintain myelin sheaths, the protective fatty coating that helps electrical signals transmit quickly and efficiently between nerve cells. Without this shielding, nerve signaling becomes disjointed, leading to a host of neurological symptoms. Researchers have connected aggressive and impulsive behaviors to a lack of myelination in the frontal lobe of the brain (Hoptman et al., 2002).

Lithium increases the uptake of vitamin B12 and folate into cells, thereby supporting myelin production. Increasing vitamin B12 and folate transport could thus be a main pathway through which lithium reduces erratic or violent behavior (Schrauzer et al., 1992).

### *Lithium Optimizes Serotonin*
As we've discussed throughout this book, serotonin is one of the key neurotransmitters, or chemical messengers, in the nervous system for managing emotional reactivity. Under normal conditions, serotonin works in the frontal areas of the brain to inhibit the firing of the amygdala, an almond-shaped structure that controls fear, anger, and other emotional responses. When serotonin levels decline, however, the amygdala becomes hyperactive, and individuals are more likely to act out in impulsive ways. Low serotonin has been linked to many behavior problems. Specifically, decreased levels of the main serotonin metabolite, called 5-hydroxyindolacetic acid (5- HIAA), have been strongly associated with aggression in humans (Brown et al., 1982; Stanley et al., 2000).

Lithium works to enhance serotonergic neurotransmission in several distinct ways. First lithium acts pre-synaptically on serotonin-sending cells to allow for more serotonin to be passed from one brain cell to another. Lithium ions then work post-synaptically, up-regulating receptors on the cells that receive the serotonin, called 5-HT1A receptors, so that they are able to collect and benefit from a greater volume. Additionally, researchers hypothesize, lithium blocks the serotonin "transporter protein" known as 5 HTT. This protein would ordinarily clear away serotonin at the synapse between the sending and receiving cells. When the transporter is blocked, excess serotonin can be taken up by the receiving cell instead (Parsey, 2009).

Lithium is therefore involved in several pathways in the serotonergic system so that it is able to properly defend the amygdala and contribute to an appropriate response to fear and anger. Serotonin is critical for appetite regulation, mood, and inhibition of the firing of the amygdala to prevent excessive fear and anger responses to minor environmental stimuli.

### *Monoamine Oxidase Activity*
Monoamine Oxidase A (MAOA) is an enzyme that degrades certain neurotransmitters in the body, including norepinepherine, dopamine, and serotonin. Relative levels of MAO A determine the concentrations of these neurotransmitters that remain present in the brain and other organs. This has a significant impact on our emotions, mood, and behavior. Monoamine oxidase activity must therefore be highly regulated to maintain a healthy mental state.

Low MAO A activity, especially in combination with experiences of childhood abuse, has been associated with an increased risk of aggressive behavior in adults (Kim-Cohen et al., 2006; Frazetto et al., 2007). Furthermore, the lower the MOA A activity in the cortical and subcortical brain regions, the higher the degree of abusive behavior. Monoamine oxidase activity appears to be directly related to the frequency and severity of aggressive behaviors (Alia-Klein et al., 2008). Lithium works to stabilize the monoamine oxidase activity, primarily through increasing MAO A activity. This is another potential pathway through which lithium could minimize aggressive behaviors in prone individuals.

## Alleviating Behavioral Aggression
It has been well-established that pharmaceutical doses of lithium have a moderating effect on aggressive and irritable behavior, as well as associated mental health disorders. However, problems with adverse effects and treatment adherence have historically prevented the widespread use of lithium.

Now, a growing body of evidence exists to support lithium's ability to mitigate these behavioral symptoms at low doses—safely and without side effects. The first compelling evidence to support the use of low-dose lithium for behavioral aggression came from environmental studies that found decreased

## Lithium as a Medicine: Irritability, Anger and Aggression

rates of mental illness as well as violent and aggressive crime in areas with lithium-rich water. Hair analyses focused on lithium levels in criminals further suggested that lithium deficiency could be a major contributing factor to aggression, and predicted that replenishing cellular stores could reverse troublesome behaviors. Based in these findings, a series of clinical trials, case studies, and biochemical investigations have demonstrated that low-dose lithium *can* decisively modify patterns of aggressive and addictive behaviors.

## CHAPTER 11 | References

Alia-Klein, N., Goldstein, R. Z., Kriplani, A., Logan, J., Tomasi, D., Williams, B., & ... Fowler, J. S. (2008). Brain monoamine oxidase A activity predicts trait aggression. *Journal of Neuroscience, 28*(19), 5099-5104.

Brown, G. L., Goodwin, F. K., & Bunney, W. J. (1982). Human aggression and suicide: their relationship to neuropsychiatric diagnoses and serotonin metabolism. *Advances in Biochemical Psychopharmacology, 34*, 287-307.

Campbell, M., Small, A. M., Green, W. H., Jennings, S. J., Perry, R., Bennett, W. G., & Anderson, L. (1984). Behavioral efficacy of haloperidol and lithium carbonate. A comparison in hospitalized aggressive children with conduct disorder. *Archives of General Psychiatry, 41*(7), 650-656.

Campbell, M., Adams, P. B., Small, A. M., Kafantaris, V., Silva, R. R., Shell, J., & ... Overall, J. E. (1995). Lithium in hospitalized aggressive children with conduct disorder: a double-blind and placebo-controlled study. *Journal of the American Academy of Child and Adolescent Psychiatry, 34*(4), 445.

Dawson, E. B., Moore, T. D., & McGanity, W. J. (1970). The mathematical relationship of drinking water lithium and rainfall to mental hospital admission. *Diseases of the Nervous System, 31*(12), 811-820.

DeLong, R. G., & Aldershof, A. L. (1987). Long-term experience with lithium treatment in childhood: Correlation with clinical diagnosis. *Journal of the American Academy of Child & Adolescent Psychiatry, 26*(3), 389-394.

Dickstein, D. P. (2015). The path to somewhere: Moving toward a better biological understanding of irritability. *American Journal of Psychiatry, 172*(7), 603-605.

de Prado-Lima, P., Knijnik, L., Juruena, M., & Padilla, A. (2001). Lithium reduces maternal child abuse behaviour: a preliminary report. *Journal of Clinical Pharmacy & Therapeutics, 26*(4), 279-282.

Ford, E. (2015). First-episode psychosis in the criminal justice system: Identifying a critical intercept for early intervention. *Harvard Review of Psychiatry, 23*(3), 167-175.

Frazzetto, G., Di Lorenzo, G., Carola, V., Proietti, L., Sokolowska, E., Siracusano, A., & ... Troisi, A. (2007). Early trauma and increased risk for physical aggression during adulthood: the moderating role of MAOA genotype. *Plos One, 2*(5), e486.

Giotakos, O., Nisianakis, P., Tsouvelas, G., & Giakalou, V.V. (2013). Lithium in the public water supply and suicide mortality in Greece. *Biological Trace Elements Research, 156*(1-3), 376-9.

Hoptman, M.J., Volavka, J., Johnson, G., Weiss, E., Bilder, R.M., &Lim, K.O. (2002) Frontal white matter microstructure, aggression, and impulsivity in men with schizophrenia: a preliminary study. *Biological Psychiatry, 52*(1):9-14.

Kabacs, N., Memon, A., Obinwa, T., Stochl, J., & Perez, J. (2011). Lithium in drinking water and suicide rates across the East of England. *British Journal of Psychiatry, 198*(5), 406-7.

Kapusta, N. D., & König, D. (2015). Naturally occurring low-dose lithium in drinking water. *Journal of Clinical Psychiatry, 76*(3), e373-e374.

Kapusta, N. D., Mossaheb, N., Etzersdorfer, E., Hlavin, G., Thau, K., Willeit, M., & ... Leithner-Dziubas, K. (2011). Lithium in drinking water and suicide mortality. *British Journal of Psychiatry, 198*(5), 346-350.

Kim-Cohen, J., Caspi, A., Taylor, A., Williams, B., Newcombe, R., Craig, I. W., & Moffitt, T. E. (2006). MAOA, maltreatment, and gene-environment interaction predicting children's mental health: New evidence and a meta-analysis. *Molecular Psychiatry, 11*(10), 903-913.

Leibenluft, E., Cohen, P., Gorrindo, T., Brook, J. S., & Pine, D. S. (2006). Chronic versus episodic irritability in youth: a community-based longitudinal study of clinical and diagnostic associations. *Journal of Child and Adolescent Psychopharmacology, 16*(4), 456-466.

Malone, R. P., Luebbert, J., Pena-Ariet, M., Biesecker, K., & Delaney, M. A. (1994). The Overt Aggression Scale in a study of lithium in aggressive conduct disorder. *Psychopharmacology Bulletin, 30*(2), 215-218.

Malone, R. P., Delaney, M. A., Leubbert, J. F., Cater, J., & Campbell, M. (2000). A double-blind placebo-controlled study of lithium in hospitalized aggressive children and adolescents with conduct disorder. *Archives of General Psychiatry, 57*(7), 649-654.

Masi, G., Milone, A., Manfredi, A., Pari, C., Paziente, A., & Millepiedi, S. (2009). Effectiveness of lithium in children and adolescents with conduct disorder: a retrospective naturalistic study. *CNS Drugs, 23*(1), 59.

Pappadopulos, E., Woolston, S., Chait, A., Perkins, M., Connor, D. F., & Jensen, P. S. (2006). Pharmacotherapy of aggression in children and adolescents: Efficacy and effect size. *Journal of the Canadian Academy of Child and Adolescent Psychiatry, 15*(1), 27-39.

Parsey, R. (2009). Understanding the mechanism of action of lithium and the pathophysiology of bipolar disorder with molecular imaging of the serotonin system. *The Dana Foundation.*

Perlis, R. H., Huang, J., Purcell, S., Fava, M., Rush, A. J., Sullivan, P. F., & ... Smoller, J. W. (2010). Genome-wide association study of suicide attempts in mood disorder patients. *American Journal of Psychiatry, 167*(12), 1499–1507.

Perou, R., Bitsko, R. H., Blumberg, S. J., Pastor, P., Ghandour, R. M., Gfroerer, J. C., & ... Huang, L. N. (2013). Mental health surveillance among children--United States, 2005-2011. *Morbidity and Mortality Weekly Report Surveillance Summaries (Washington, D.C.: 2002), 62*(Suppl 2), 1-35.

Peterson, B. S., Zhang, H., Santa Lucia, R., King, R. A., & Lewis, M. (1996). Risk factors for presenting problems in child psychiatric emergencies. *Journal Of The American Academy Of Child And Adolescent Psychiatry, 35*(9), 1162–1173.

Tupin, J. P., Smith, D. B., Clanon, T. L., Kim, L. I., Nugent, A., & Groupe, A. (1973). The long-term use of lithium in aggressive prisoners. *Comprehensive Psychiatry, 14*(4), 311-317.

Roberson-Nay, R., Leibenluft, E., Brotman, M. A., Myers, J., Larsson, H., Lichtenstein, P., & Kendler, K. S. (2015). Longitudinal stability of genetic and environmental influences on irritability: From childhood to young adulthood. *American Journal of Psychiatry, 172*(7), 657-664.

Schrauzer, G. N., & deVroey, E. (1994). Effects of nutritional lithium supplementation on mood. A placebo-controlled study with former drug users. *Biological Trace Element Research, 40*(1), 89-101.

Schrauzer, G.N. & Shrestha, K.P. (1990). Lithium in drinking water and the incidences of crimes, suicides, and arrests related to drug addictions. *Biological Trace Elements Research, 25*(2), 105-13.

Schrauzer, G. N., Shrestha, K. P., & Flores-Arce, M. F. (1992). Lithium in scalp hair of adults, students, and violent criminals. Effects of supplementation and evidence for interactions of lithium with vitamin B12 and with other trace elements. *Biological Trace Element Research, 34*(2), 161-176.

Sheard, M. H. (1975). Lithium in the treatment of aggression. *Journal of Nervous and Mental Disease, 160*(2), 108-118.

Sheard, M. H., Marini, J. L., Bridges, C. I., & Wagner, E. (1976). The effect of lithium on impulsive aggressive behavior in man. *American Journal of Psychiatry, 133*(12), 1409-1413.

Snaith, R. P., & Taylor, C. M. (1985). Irritability: Definition, Assessment and Associated Factors. *British Journal of Psychiatry, 147,* 127.

Stanley, B, Molcho, A, Stanley, M, Winchel, R, Gameroff, M J, Parsons, B, & Mann, J J. (2000). Association of aggressive behavior with altered serotonergic function in patients who are not suicidal. *American Journal of Psychiatry, 157*(4), 609-14.

Stringaris, A., Cohen, P., Pine, D. S., & Leibenluft, E. (2009). Adult outcomes of youth irritability: a 20-year prospective community-based study. *American Journal of Psychiatry, 166*(9),1048.

Sugawara, N., Yasui-Furukori, N., Ishii, N., Iwata, N., & Terao, T. (2013). Lithium in tap water and suicide mortality in Japan. *International Journal of Environmental Research and Public Health, 10*(11), 6044-6048.

# Twelve

## LITHIUM AS A MEDICINE: ADDICTION AND SUBSTANCE ABUSE

At least 23 million Americans age 12 and older have substance use disorders. Globally, alcohol misuse is the fifth leading risk factor for premature death and disability; among people between the ages of 15 and 49, it is the first. The use of illicit drugs has increased over the last decade from 8.3% of the population using in 2002, to 9.4% in 2013. Sadly, of all the individuals struggling with substance use disorders, only about 11% will receive treatment the treatment they need this year (SAMSHA, 2015; NIAAA, 2015).

Substance use disorders are a growing public health concern. These pervasive disorders occur when the repetitive use of alcohol and/or drugs causes clinically significant impairment, including health problems, disability, and a failure to meet major responsibilities at work, school, or home. Abuse of tobacco, alcohol, and illicit drugs is destructive to communities and families, and also costly to our nation, demanding more than $700 billion annually due to crime, lost work productivity, and health care (NIDA, 2015).

Substance use disorders affect individuals across population groups. However, people with mental health issues are at a markedly higher risk for experiencing alcohol or substance use problems than those not affected by mental illness. Compared with the general population, people addicted to drugs

## Lithium as a Medicine: Addiction and Substance Abuse

are twice as likely to suffer from mood and anxiety disorders; the reverse is also true. Three large epidemiological studies conducted over the last 25 years have confirmed that there is a high prevalence of substance abuse among those with mental illnesses, particularly individuals with mood disorders (Tolliver & Anoton, 2015).

According to the National Institute on Drug Abuse (NIDA), there are common biological, psychological, and social risk factors that may influence the simultaneous appearance of substance use and mental illness. These include:

- Genetic vulnerability. Certain genetic predispositions may make an individual more susceptible to addictive behaviors and mental health disorders, or place them at greater risk for developing the second once one occurs.
- Environmental triggers. Stress, trauma, and early exposure to drugs are prominent environmental factors impacting addiction and other mental illnesses.
- Involvement of similar brain regions. The brain systems responsible for managing reward and stress can be abnormal in patients with mental health disorders, and are also altered by drugs of abuse.
- Drug use disorders and other mental illnesses are developmental disorders. Both frequently begin in teenage years or younger, during periods when the nervous system is undergoing rapid developmental changes. Early exposure to drugs of abuse may change the brain in ways that increase the risk for mental disorders, while early symptoms of a mental disorder may indicate an increased risk for later drug use (NIDA, 2011).

The recurrence of symptoms and behaviors in individuals with addiction and other substance use disorders is similar to relapse rates for well-understood chronic medical illnesses such as diabetes, hypertension, and asthma (NIDA, 2014). This suggests that addiction and substance abuse should be treated and managed with the same degree of specialized medical care and attention as other chronic illnesses. The consequences of untreated or undertreated co-occurring mental health and substance disorders are dire, including a higher likelihood that the patient will experience homelessness, incarceration, medical illness, suicide, and early death (SAMSHA, 2015).

In order for addiction treatment to be successful, therapies must be tailored to the needs of the individual and based on personal circumstances and goals. Integrated treatment strategies that occur across a variety of disciplines and settings have been found to be the most effective. Evidence demonstrates that beneficial long-term results are best achieved when a combination of individual and group counseling, medication, and community support services are accessed. Other strategies such as nutritional supplementation, acupuncture, yoga, and mindfulness have also proven useful. Overall, treatments that address mental health and substance abuse conditions at the same time rather than sequentially are associated with lower cost and better outcomes including reduced substance use, improved psychiatric symptoms, decreased hospitalization, increased housing stability, fewer arrests, and improved quality of life.

One therapeutic strategy that has proven extremely useful for treating addiction and substance use is supplementation with the mineral lithium. A significant literature demonstrates that pharmaceutical lithium can attenuate addictive patterning, and a smaller group of studies have suggested that lithium deficiency could possibly contribute to addictive behaviors.

## Genetics and Reward Deficiency Syndrome

Although there is no alcoholism gene or strict cause-and-effect relationship between genetics and behavior, there are aspects of human behavior associated with particular genes. Beginning in the early 1990s, researchers became interested in a specific genetic anomaly that was linked to alcoholism. Later research found that this genetic anomaly is also found with increased frequency among people with other addictive or impulsive disorders, including substance abuse, smoking, compulsive overeating, obesity, attention-deficit disorder, Tourette's syndrome, and pathological gambling (Blum et al., 1996).

# Lithium as a Medicine: Addiction and Substance Abuse

An aberration of any of the genes involved in the brain's reward pathway may predispose an individual to alcoholism. In 1972, it was discovered that adopted children whose biological parents were alcoholics were more likely to have a drinking problem than those born to nonalcoholic parents. Likewise, a year later it was discovered that sons born to alcoholic fathers were three times more likely to become alcoholic than the sons of nonalcoholic fathers (Blum et al., 1996).

Kenneth Blum has coined the term "reward deficiency syndrome" to explain how a seemingly simple genetic abnormality could led to a complex deviant behavior. "This syndrome involves a form of sensory deprivation of the brain's pleasure mechanisms. It can be manifested in relatively mild or severe forms that follow as a consequence of an individual's biochemical inability to derive reward from ordinary, everyday activities." The chemical imbalance alters signaling in the brain's reward process and replaces feelings of well-being with anxiety, anger, or a craving for a substance that can alleviate the negative emotions. The same genetic variant associated with alcoholism leads to an alteration in the reward pathways of the brain. Specifically, it is a variant form of the gene for the dopamine D2 receptor called the A1 allele (Blum et al., 1996).

Most addictions, including alcohol, opiates, cocaine, methamphetamine, nicotine, carbohydrates, gambling, and sex addiction, are associated with the release of dopamine in the reward pathway of the brain. When the dopaminergic system is activated, one has feelings of reward and pleasure. Reduced dopaminergic activity can trigger drug-seeking behavior in hopes to achieving those feelings of pleasure (Blum et al., 2012).

This abnormal dopamine receptor gene is often altered in cocaine addicts. About 52 percent of cocaine addicts have the A1 allele of the dopamine D2 receptor gene, compared to only 21 percent of nonaddicts. In fact, the prevalence of the allele rises to almost 90 percent when the addict has three certain risk factors: parental alcoholism and drug abuse, strong cocaine potency, and early-childhood deviant behavior (Blum et al., 1996).

There is a similarity between the euphoric state of the gambler and the "high" of the substance abuser. Like drug abusers, pathological gamblers develop tolerance; they need to take greater risks and make larger bets to reach a desired level of excitement. They experience withdrawal-like symptoms. Again, the dopamine brain pathways may be involved with pathological gambling. A study of pathological gamblers found that 51 percent carried the A1 allele of the dopamine D2 receptor. There was a higher likelihood of carrying the A1 allele the more severe the gambling problem. In a group of pathological gambling males with drug problems, the incidence of the A1 allele rose to almost 80 percent (Blum et al., 1996).

## Lithium, Mood, and Impulse Control

It is most commonly hypothesized that lithium catalyzes changes in addictive behaviors primarily by lessening underlying impulsivity, irritability, and volatile mood. As described above, several studies have reported a strong association between alcoholism, drug abuse, and mood disorders. To date, there have been two large epidemiological studies on the subject, demonstrating that between 30-60% of those with affective disorders have a concurrent substance use disorder (Sonne & Brady, 2002).

There is substantial evidence to suggest that lithium is most effective for treating comorbid substance use disorders because it modifies the irritable mood states and impulsive behaviors that drive the use of alcohol and drugs. For individuals with bipolar disorder, for example, substance abuse most commonly occurs during the manic phase of the disorder or the period in which patients experience an abnormally elevated, expansive, or irritable mood. Because lithium can be used to stabilize this state of hyperarousal, it possibly has the indirect effect of preventing excessive alcohol and drug use during this vulnerable time. Lithium has also been shown to decrease generalized irritability and pathological impulsive aggression independently, both of which are believed to be key features of the "alcoholic personality" (McMillan, 1981).

Previous studies have found a significant inverse correlation between drug-related crimes and the lithium concentration of drinking water. This suggests that those who are deficient in lithium could have a lower threshold for developing drug dependency. A double-blind placebo-controlled experiment involving nutritional lithium supplementation (1/1000 of the therapeutic dose) was conducted with former users of stimulant drugs (e.g., cocaine, heroin, crystal methamphetamine). In the lithium group, mood improvement was statistically significant after only one week of lithium supplementation and remained so throughout the trial. Every single subject who took lithium experienced an enhanced mood, specifically in measures of happiness, friendliness, and energy. The placebo group did not experience any consistent mood changes (Schrauzer & de Vroey, 1994).

## Lithium for Relapse Prevention

Five double-blind placebo controlled studies have investigated the use of pharmaceutical-dose lithium as a direct relapse preventative in alcoholic patients (Kline et al., 1974; Merry et al., 1976; Clark & Fawcett, 1989; Fawcett et al., 2000; Dorus et al., 1989). Of these studies, however, only three have managed to keep substantial levels of participants in treatment long enough to yield significant results.

The first lasted for two years and followed 73 detoxified chronic alcoholics. The treatment group was given a daily dose of lithium carbonate, while the other subjects received a placebo. All other medications in both groups were discontinued for one month prior to the start of the study. Over the research period, substantially fewer drinking episodes were reported in the lithium group compared to the placebo group and when compared to their own frequency of drinking in years prior to the study. After 48 weeks, relapses occurred in nine of 14 patients on placebo as compared to just four of 16 in the lithium group. Bouts of drinking were both less severe and of shorter duration in those given lithium (Kline et al., 1974).

Another study reviewing lithium as a relapse preventative followed 71 alcoholics who had undergone detoxification. Patients were classified as depressed or non-depressed and randomly assigned to receive either lithium carbonate or a placebo. Changes in alcoholic morbidity were assessed based on the number of reported days subjects spent incapacitated by alcohol. Lithium reduced episodes of drinking in depressed alcoholics as compared to the placebo group, but there was no significant difference in the non-depressed groups. Authors of this study suggested that lithium's effects on reducing drinking behaviors in alcoholic patients do involve changes in mood state, although the specific nature of this relationship is unclear (Merry et al., 1976).

Lithium has thus been found to be superior to placebo in preventing relapse in alcoholics, particularly for those also struggling with depression. Further double-blind study is required, however, as several gaps exist within the current literature. First, treatment adherence posed a major complication in almost every trial, with retention rates around 50% or less. While studies following substance abusers typically have low retention rates, understanding the circumstances and characteristics of drop-outs would help to determine if individuals left the studies because they were treatment failures, non-responders, or had undesirable side effects. Additional research is needed to determine whether or not the relapse-preventing effects of lithium are due to its mood-stabilizing qualities, or if there are other mechanisms at work directly related to addiction and the brain-reward pathways.

## Lithium & Alcohol Conditioning

There are several studies indicating that the therapeutic effects of lithium on substance users are not simply the result of alleviating associated affective symptoms. Lithium may indeed have other mechanisms for decreasing addictive behaviors that are not directly related to mood.

One pharmacological strategy for minimizing substance abuse is to administer a medication that induces negative feelings when a substance is taken. The most common medication among this group is disulfiram (Antabuse), which produces unpleasant effects when even small amounts of alcohol are consumed. These effects begin about 10 minutes after alcohol enters the body and include flushing of the face, headache, nausea, vomiting, chest pain, weakness, blurred vision, mental confusion, sweating, choking, breathing difficulty, and anxiety. Medications like disulfiram clearly discourage drinking and for some act as a powerful deterrent to more consumption.

# Lithium as a Medicine: Addiction and Substance Abuse

Lithium was used to successfully produce this kind of conditioned aversion in animals, and these effects have now been studied in humans as well. In one study, 25 detoxified alcoholics were given relatively high doses of oral lithium. Subjects taking the lithium reported that alcohol produced symptoms similar to a 'hangover' and in 67% of cases, these sickness reactions were considered of sufficient intensity to halt the behavior. At the six-month follow-up, 36% of the lithium-treated group remained abstinent, a significant result as compared to controls. The authors also noted that no medical complications occurred during the acute period of lithium administration nor during the six-month follow-up period, even though high doses were being used (Boland, Mellor, & Revusky, 1978). These data suggest that lithium is indeed a safe treatment for this population group.

## Lithium Reduces Drug-Induced Euphoria

Lithium has been shown to decrease drug-induced euphoria in drug abusers in at least eight studies (McMillan, 1981). This means that lithium has the potential to alter the body's response to a substance so that it no longer evokes the same desirable "high." Medications with this quality can lessen cravings and help the brain to adapt gradually to the absence of the abused drug. In one double-blind study on the subject, 27 chronic alcoholics were given alcohol after detoxification (Judd et al., 1979). Lithium was then administered for 14 days, and its effects on a variety of cognitive tests were compared to placebo. Euphoric effects were not blocked completely, but were reduced by lithium. Individuals with a past history of major depressive disorders experienced the most significant response to lithium. Yet high drop-out rates, likely due to the side effects of high doses, have remained problematic in drawing clear study conclusions from these types of studies.

Lithium shows promise in the treatment of amphetamine addiction. In the first documented report, two amphetamine abusers spontaneously gave up the drug because they lost the "high" feeling after starting lithium treatment for affective disorders (Flemenbaum, 1974). A double-blind, placebo-controlled trial of amphetamine was conducted with moderately to severely depressed patients. Treatment with lithium carbonate produced a 60% attenuation of euphoria responses to dextroamphetamine. The responses to levoamphetamine were almost completely abolished by lithium (Van Kammen & Murphy, 1975). In an open trial of eight psychiatric hospital patients, approximately half showed some attenuation of the stimulant effects of amphetamine after pretreatment with lithium. Two showed specific blockade of euphoria (Angrist, & Gershon, 1979). A double-blind crossover trial revealed that lithium alone caused a decreased sense of "high" from the stimulant methylphenidate (Huey et al., 1981).

There is potential for lithium treatment in cocaine abuse. Lithium and cocaine seem to have opposing effects on regulating serotonin 5-HT synthesis. Lithium enhances the conversion of tryptophan to 5-HT. In rats, cocaine hydrochloride inhibits the uptake of tryptophan, reducing its conversion to 5-HT. When researchers injected cocaine hydrochloride into rats after three days of lithium injections, there were no apparent effects on the 5-HT system. Lithium protected the serotonergic neurons against the usual effects of cocaine (Mandell & Knapp, 1976). Longitudinal observation of long-term cocaine users supports the use of lithium in cyclothymic-bipolar patients. Cyclothymic subjects who were given lithium stopped their cocaine use and remained cocaine-free for more than three months. In these patients, cocaine use stopped abruptly after lithium administration was started (Gawin & Kleber, 1984). Multiple case studies have clearly demonstrated blockade of cocaine euphoria by lithium (Cronson & Flemenbaum, 1978; Gold & Byck, 1978).

## Lithium for Gambling Addiction

Pathological gambling is classified as an addictive disorder in DSM-V. Pathological gambling often goes undiagnosed, and there is currently no FDA-approved treatment. It is a serious social issue, as people with this condition have attempted suicide rates as high as 20%. Lithium may reduce addiction severity in pathological gamblers (Chaim et al., 2014).

In one randomized study, after 14 weeks of lithium treatment, subjects with severe addictive gambling behaviors showed a significant improvement in pathological gambling symptoms (Pallanti et al., 2002). Significant improvements were seen after just four weeks.

A 10-week randomized double-blind trial compared sustained-release lithium to placebo in 40 patients with bipolar disorder. Significant differences were seen between the lithium group and placebo group in gambling behavior and thoughts, with the lithium group having less severe thoughts, urges, and gambling behavior by the end of the study. The mood-stabilizing effects of lithium may reduce rapid mood swings associated with energized activity, urgency, and faster decision making (Hollander et al., 2005).

Chaim et al. (2014) presented a recent case study of a 42-year-old pathological gambler with a history of substance abuse disorder, including alcohol and cocaine, and increased sexual appetite. The patient was given lithium and monitored for 18 months. At his first follow-up, his mood was more stable and he was less irritable than he had been before the study began. He had greater self-control over gambling with decreased stakes and began to pay his debts. At his second follow-up, he had remission of gambling behaviors and maintained the less irritable mood, a change verified by others.

## Modifying Addictive Behaviors with Lithium

Affective disorders and substance use disorders are widespread in the general population, and their co-occurrence is common. It has been estimated, for example, that between 30-60% of alcoholics struggle with depression and a comparable percentage of depressed patients also have a substance abuse disorder. There are many reasons to explain this overlap, including shared genetic, environmental, biological, and developmental risk factors.

The treatment of co-occurring substance use disorders and mental illness can be difficult and often requires the layering of many different approaches and techniques. Individual and group counseling, community support, and medication have all proven useful for managing substances use, as have integrative therapies such as yoga, acupuncture, and nutritional support. One key strategy is the use of lithium, which even at low doses has shown profound effects on the human brain.

## Nutritional Lithium: A Cinderella Story

Lithium can help to mediate the underlying irritability, aggression, and mood instability that often drive addictive behaviors. Additional research is needed to clarify whether lithium can treat substance abuse independently of modulating mood. Some studies have suggested that lithium can be used as a conditioning agent to discourage drinking by spurring a negative physical reaction when alcohol is consumed. Other researchers have demonstrated that lithium can decrease the euphoric effects of drugs, making them less sought-after. It is possible that lithium works through all of these pathways, thus providing multiple layers of benefits to patients working towards recovery.

Low-dose lithium has emerged as a promising treatment option for those with a personal or family history of substance abuse. There is fascinating epidemiological and clinical evidence to show that small doses of lithium may help to restore optimal brain health and shift addictive patterns in a manner that is both safe and effective.

## CHAPTER 12 | References

Angrist, B., & Gershon, S. (1979). Variable attenuation of amphetamine effects by lithium. *American Journal of Psychiatry, 136*(6), 806-810.

Blum, K., Cull, J. G., Braverman, E. R., & Comings, D. E. (1996). Reward Deficiency Syndrome. *American Scientist, 84*(2), 132–145.

Blum, K., Oscar-Berman, M., Giordano, J., Downs, B., Simpatico, T., Han, D., & Femino, J. (2012). Neurogenetic Impairments of Brain Reward Circuitry Links to Reward Deficiency Syndrome (RDS): Potential Nutrigenomic Induced Dopaminergic Activation. *Journal of Genetic Syndromes & Gene Therapy, 3*(4), 1000e115.

Boland, F. J., Mellor, C. S., & Revusky, S. (1978). Chemical aversion treatment of alcoholism: Lithium as the aversive agent. *Behaviour Research and Therapy, 16*(6), 401-409.

Chaim, C. H., Nazar, B. P., Hollander, E., & Lessa, J. M. (2014). Pathological gambling treated with lithium: The role of assessing temperament. *Addictive Behaviors, 39*(12), 1911-1913.

Clark, D. C., & Fawcett, J. (1989). Does lithium carbonate therapy for alcoholism deter relapse drinking? *Recent Developments in Alcoholism, 7*, 315-328.

Cronson, A. J., & Flemenbaum, A. (1978). Antagonism of cocaine highs by lithium. *American Journal of Psychiatry, 135*(7), 856-857.

Dawson, E. B., Moore, T. D., & McGanity, W. J. (1970). The mathematical relationship of drinking water lithium and rainfall to mental hospital admission. *Diseases of the Nervous System, 31*(12), 811-820.

Dorus, W., Ostrow, D. G., Anton, R., Cushman, P., Collins, J. F., Schaefer, M., & ... Sather, M. R. (1989). Lithium treatment of depressed and nondepressed alcoholics. *JAMA, 262*(12), 1646-52.

Fawcett, J., Kravitz, H. M., McGuire, M., Easton, M., Ross, J., Pisani, V., & ... Teas, G. (2000). Pharmacological treatments for alcoholism: Revisiting lithium and considering buspirone. *Alcoholism: Clinical and Experimental Research, 24*(5), 666-674.

Flemenbaum, A. (1974). Does lithium block the effects of amphetamine? A report of three cases. *American Journal of Psychiatry, 131*(7), 820-1.

Gawin, F. H., & Kleber, H. D. (1984). Cocaine abuse treatment: Open pilot trial with desipramine and lithium carbonate. *Archives of General Psychiatry, 41*(9), 903-909.

Geller, B., Cooper, T. B., Sun, K., Zimerman, B., Frazier, J., Williams, M., & Heath, J. (1998). Double-blind and placebo-controlled study of lithium for adolescent bipolar disorders with secondary substance dependency. *Journal of the American Academy of Child and Adolescent Psychiatry, 37*(2), 171.

Giotakos, O., Nisianakis, P., Tsouvelas, G., & Giakalou, V.V. (2013). Lithium in the public water supply and suicide mortality in Greece. *Biological Trace Elements Research, 156*(1-3), 376-9.

Gold, M. S., & Byck, R. (1978). Endorphins, lithium, and naloxone: their relationship to pathological and drug-induced manic-euphoric states. *NIDA Research Monograph*, (19), 192-209.

Hollander, E., Pallanti, S., Allen, A., Sood, E., & Rossi, N. (2005). Does sustained-release lithium reduce impulsive gambling and affective instability versus placebo in pathological gamblers with bipolar spectrum disorders? *American Journal of Psychiatry, 162*(1), 137-145.

Huey, L., Janowsky, D., Judd, L., Abrams, A., Parker, D., & Clopton, P. (1981). Effects of lithium carbonate on methylphenidate-induced mood, behavior, and cognitive processes. *Psychopharmacology, 73*(2), 161.

Judd, L. L., et al. (1979). Ethanol-lithium interaction in alcoholics. In: D. W. Goodwin and C. K. Erikson (eds), *Alcoholism and Affective Disorders*, New York, NY: Spectrum, pp. 109-135.

Kapusta, N. D., Mossaheb, N., Etzersdorfer, E., et al. (2011). Lithium in drinking water and suicide mortality. *British Journal of Psychiatry, 198*(5), 346-350.

Kline, N. S., Wren, J. C., Cooper, T. B., Varga, E., & Canal, O. (1974). Evaluation of lithium therapy in chronic and periodic alcoholism. *American Journal of the Medical Sciences, 268*(1), 15-22.

Mandell, A., & Knapp, S. (1976). A Neurobiological Model for the Symmetrical Prophylactic Action of Lithium in Bipolar Affective Disorder. *Pharmakopsychiatrie, Neuro-Psychopharmakologie, 9*(3), 116.

McMillan, T. (1981). Lithium and the Treatment of Alcoholism: A Critical Review. *British Journal of Addiction, 76*(2), 245-258.

Merry, J., Reynolds, C. M., Bailey, J., & Coppen, A. (1976). Prophylactic treatment of alcoholism by lithium carbonate. A controlled study. *Lancet, 1*(7984), 481-482.

National Institute on Alcohol Abuse and Alcoholism (NIAAA). (2015). *Alcohol facts and statistics.* Retrieved from www.niaaa.nih.gov/alcohol-health/overview-alcohol-consumption/alcohol-facts-and-statistics

National Institute on Drug Abuse (NIDA). (2011). *DrugFacts: Comorbidity: Addiction and Other Mental Health Disorders.* National Institutes of Health. Retrieved from www.drugabuse.gov/publications/drugfacts/comorbidity-addiction-other-mental-disorders

National Institute on Drug Abuse (NIDA). (2014). *Drugs, Brains, and Behavior: The Science of Addiction.* National Institutes of Health. Retrieved from www.drugabuse.gov/publications/drugs-brains-behavior-science-addiction/treatment-recovery

National Institute on Drug Abuse (NIDA). (2015). *Trends and statistics.* National Institutes of Health. Retrieved from www.drugabuse.gov/related-topics/trends-statistics

Pallanti, S., Quercioli, L., Sood, E., & Hollander, E. (2002). Lithium and valproate treatment of pathological gambling: a randomized single-blind study. *Journal of Clinical Psychiatry, 63*(7), 559-564.

Schrauzer, G. N., & deVroey, E. (1994). Effects of nutritional lithium supplementation on mood. A placebo-controlled study with former drug users. *Biological Trace Element Research, 40*(1), 89-101.

Schrauzer, G.N. & Shrestha, K.P. (1990). Lithium in drinking water and the incidences of crimes, suicides, and arrests related to drug addictions. *Biological Trace Elements Research, 25*(2), 105-13.

Sonne, S., & Brady, K. (2002). Bipolar disorder and alcoholism. *Alcohol Research & Health, 26*(2), 103-108.

Sugawara, N., Yasui-Furukori, N., Ishii, N., Iwata, N., & Terao, T. (2013). Lithium in tap water and suicide mortality in Japan. *International Journal of Environmental Research and Public Health, 10*(11), 6044-6048.

Substances Abuse and Mental Health Service Administration (SAMSHA). (2015). *Alcohol, tobacco and other drugs*. Retrieved from www.samhsa.gov/topics/alcohol-tobacco-other-drugs

Tolliver, B. K., & Anton, R. F. (2015). Assessment and treatment of mood disorders in the context of substance abuse. *Dialogues in Clinical Neuroscience, 17*(2), 181-190.

Van Kammen, D. P., & Murphy, D. L. (1975). Attenuation of the euphoriant and activating effects of d- and l-amphetamine by lithium carbonate treatment. *Psychopharmacologia, 44*(3), 215-224.

# Thirteen

## LITHIUM AS A MEDICINE: EATING DISORDERS AND ATTENTION-DEFICIT HYPERACTIVITY DISORDER

Lithium is approved by the U.S. Food and Drug Administration for its mood stabilizing effects in bipolar disorder treatment, but its clinical uses now span a number of neuropsychiatric conditions. As we have covered in previous chapters, lithium salts have been used to resolve mental health disorders as diverse as depression, aggression, irritability, and addiction, as well as related neurodegenerative disorders. The biological theory underscoring these successes is that lithium reduces neuronal excitability, restores neurochemical balance, and encourages regeneration of damaged brain tissue. These features have also made lithium of interest in my work with eating disorder patients and those with ADHD. In both of these disorders, impulse control and mood regulation also play an important role. In this chapter we will review the research suggesting lithium as a logical, albeit underused, treatment for eating disorders and ADHD.

## Eating Disorders

Research studies have demonstrated that lithium may have positive effects on patients with eating disorders. Eating disorders are characterized by an

# Nutritional Lithium: A Cinderella Story

obsession with food, body image, and weight. The disorders cause disturbances to everyday diet, such as restricting food or severely overeating, which can become serious, chronic, and potentially life-threatening.

Another common feature in eating disorder patients is mood instability. In fact, multiple studies have identified an overlap between mood disorder symptoms and eating disorder behaviors. One team of researchers found that a diagnosis of bipolar II disorder was present in 59% of eating disorder inpatients (McElroy, Kotwal, & Malhotra, 2004). What's more, the co-occurrence of the disorders was associated with negative effects on the course, outcome, and response to treatment.

The relationship between mood disorders and dysfunctional eating appears consistent across different types of eating disorders. As many as half of all patients diagnosed with binge eating disorder have a history of depression, according to the National Institute of Diabetes and Digestive and Kidney Diseases (NIDDK, 2012). Mood disorders also plague many people with anorexia and bulimia; studies show that anorexics are 50 times more likely than the general population to die as a result of suicide (Arcelus et al., 2011).

The connection between mood disorders and eating disorders thus has huge clinical and theoretical significance. The reason behind their co-occurrence is not always clear: evidence exists to suggest both that mood instability can drive eating disorder behaviors, and that the malnourishment that results from abnormal food intake can spur problems with mood. Nonetheless, lithium has proven helpful for treating eating disorder symptoms of various forms and etiology, as well as concurrent mood-related symptoms.

## *Anorexia Nervosa*

Anorexia nervosa is a type of eating disorder defined by self-starvation and excessive weight loss. The first evidence suggesting lithium as a treatment for anorexia came from a small case study of two patients. After 12 weeks of lithium monotherapy, one female patient gained 26 pounds, while a second patient gained about 20 pounds after just six weeks treatment. The substantial weight gain experienced by both patients was accompanied by increased food intake as well as improved mood and capacity for work. The dose used in these patients was the pharmacological dose of 1,500 mg per day of lithium carbonate (Barcai, 1977).

A follow-up study completed a few years later evaluated the use of lithium in eight patients with anorexia nervosa. In this randomized double-blind placebo-controlled trial, patients who were treated with lithium showed greater weight gain after three and four weeks of treatment than patients receiving placebo. Lithium treatment also led to a significantly greater improvement on rating scales that measure denial of illness (Gross et al., 1981). This is important, as patients who deny their illness are not motivated to engage with therapy, and chances of recovery remain low. Reducing denial is thus an important marker for successful outcomes in eating disorder treatment.

In another more recent case study of a 25-year-old female, lithium resolved anorexia nervosa and bipolar symptoms twice. After treatment with lithium, the patient became less agitated and more rational, and did not fear gaining weight. She gained 7.7 pounds over eight days. The patient gained an additional six pounds over six weeks, but then stopped taking lithium because she thought it was unnecessary. Within several weeks symptoms of mania and depression returned, as did an obsession with being fat. Lithium treatment was initiated again, and within 10 days her symptoms subsided (Rubenstein, 1991).

## *Bulimia Nervosa*

Patients with bulimia nervosa engage in a cycle of bingeing followed by compensatory behaviors such as self-induced vomiting or extreme exercise. There has only been one open trial study on the use of lithium for bulimic patients, but results were promising. Lithium reduced bulimic episodes in 12 of 14 women involved in the study. The number of bulimic episodes was reduced by 75% to 100% in these patients. Researchers predicted that lithium addressed the patients' mood swings and emotional instability, thus leading to a decrease in bingeing and purging behaviors (Hsu, 1984).

## *Binge Eating Disorder*

Binge eating disorder is defined by recurrent episodes of eating large amounts of food, feeling a loss of control during the binge, and experiencing intense feelings of guilt and shame afterwards. Literature on lithium in binge eating disorder is also limited. One study described the successful lithium augmentation of topiramate in patients with bipolar disorder and comorbid binge eating disorder. The addition of lithium to topiramate caused 67% of patients to show improvement in both mood symptoms and weight loss. Binge eating symptoms and weekly binge frequency were both decreased after lithium augmentation. A total of 83% of participants experienced continual weight loss and reversal of resistance to weight loss or weight gain. Again, mood stabilization may have influenced remediation of binge eating symptoms (Kotwal et al., 2006).

Lithium thus appears to be a viable option to consider in addressing the symptomatology of eating disorder behaviors, especially when mood fluctuation also plays a role. It is encouraging that in all present studies with eating disorder patients, pharmacological lithium has been well tolerated and without reports of serious side effects. Low-dose lithium remains unexplored in studies with eating disorder patients, but is an important treatment to consider. Low-dose lithium has been shown to address issues of impulse control and depressed mood in studies of other disorders, and it stands to reason that these effects would be transferrable to eating disorder patents as well. This has certainly been the case at my clinic. Future studies should aim to assess the prevalence of lithium deficiency among eating disorder patients as well, to determine if a lack of this essential element may contribute to symptom development.

## Attention-Deficient Hyperactivity Disorder (ADHD)

Attention deficit hyperactivity disorder (ADHD) is one of the most common childhood disorders. It can continue through adolescence and into adulthood. ADHD affects 11% of American children 4 to 17 years old and about 4.1% of American adults aged 18 and older (CDC, 2015). ADHD is one of the top reasons for referral to a pediatrician, family physician, child psychiatrist, or psychologist (Grohol, 2014). Studies show that the number of children being diagnosed with ADHD is increasing (NIMH, n.d.).

For both children and adults, symptoms create problems at school, at work, and in relationships. Experts have linked ADHD with an increased risk of accidents, drug abuse, failure at school, antisocial behavior, and criminal activity (Grohol, 2014). Compared to children without ADHD, children with ADHD are more likely to have major injuries or hospital admission through an inpatient or outpatient programs or the emergency department (CDC, 2015).

ADHD is classified as a neurodevelopmental disorder or an impairment of the growth and development of the brain. The primary characteristics of ADHD are persistent inattention, hyperactivity, and impulsivity that interfere with functioning or a child's development. Researchers have identified several anatomical abnormalities associated with ADHD. One study found that children with ADHD had 3-4% smaller brain volumes than normal children in all brain regions measured. In particular, the brains of ADHD patients had a significantly lower amount of white matter, the type of brain tissue that helps make long-distance connections between brain regions (Grohol, 2014). Other studies have found that ADHD patients have a higher rate of resting activity in areas of the brain that process sensory stimuli (Tian et al., 2008: Qui, 2010). Atypical neurogenesis and neuronal excitability may thus be involved in ADHD pathophysiology. Together, these findings could provide a biological explanation for the impulse control and hyperactivity symptoms seen in ADHD. If this is in fact the case, lithium's neurotrophic qualities could be extremely helpful in providing relief from symptoms.

Lithium's effect on ADHD symptoms has been examined in a few studies. One 18-week randomized, double-blind study compared lithium up to 1,200 mg/day with the stimulant methylphenidate (Ritalin) up to 40 mg/day in 32 adults. Patients took the first medication for eight weeks, then had a two week washout period, followed by eight weeks on the second treatment. Both therapies led to significant improvements in irritability, aggressive outbursts, antisocial behavior, anxiety, and depression as well as significant improvements on scales of hyperactivity, impulsivity, and learning disorders (Dorrego, 2002).

An earlier study assessed the efficacy of methylphenidate and/or lithium in seven psychiatrically hospitalized prepubescent children. There was a significant improvement in hyperactivity and inattention when lithium and methylphenidate were combined (Carlson, 1992).

Pediatric bipolar disorder and ADHD share many of the same symptoms, so it is not surprising that lithium is also helpful for ADHD. ADHD may be misdiagnosed as bipolar disorder, especially in adolescents and children. Those with bipolar disorder may present with increased activity, poor concentration, increased impulsivity, or inattention. Like patients with bipolar disorder, children with ADHD may show significant changes in mood within the same day. Symptoms of mania and ADHD both include rapid speech, racing thoughts, distractibility, and less need for sleep, suggesting that they may share a common pathophysiology (APA, 2013).

Combining this evidence, it seems that lithium could prove helpful in treating symptoms of ADHD, mainly by reducing impulsivity. Lithium may also work as a CNS depressant to calm hyperactivity, reduce aggression, and improve sleep in ADHD patients. More research is needed to determine if the lithium could be useful in addressing the underlying the structural and functional abnormalities that are common in ADHD as well.

## Relief for Eating Disorders and ADHD

The mineral lithium has wide-ranging effects in psychiatry. It has been well established in the literature that lithium helps to stabilize mood and improve impulse control in patients with affective disorders. Lithium may therefore also be of benefit to individuals struggling with eating disorders and ADHD, two conditions that feature similar clinical symptoms. Preliminary research into the use of lithium in eating disorders has shown that the mineral may help to reduce dysfunctional behaviors around food and exercise, encourage normalized weight, and advance focus on recovery. In patients with ADHD, lithium has led to improvements in irritability, aggressive outbursts, hyperactivity and learning issues. I have found nutritional lithium to be one of the most important treatments available for ADHD children with impulsivity and aggression. These patients also tend to have a family history of substance abuse or mood disorders. Future studies should also examine whether deficiency of lithium, an essential element for neurological health, contributes to the pathophysiology of these connected psychiatric disorders.

## CHAPTER 13 | References

American Psychiatric Association (APA). (2013). *Diagnostic and statistical manual of mental disorders: DSM-5*. Washington, D.C: American Psychiatric Publishing.

Arcelus, J., Mitchell, A. J., Wales, J., & Nielsen, S. (2011). Mortality rates in patients with anorexia nervosa and other eating disorders: A meta-analysis of 36 studies. *Archives of General Psychiatry, 68*(7), 724-731.

Barcai, A. (1977). Lithium in adult anorexia nervosa: A pilot report on two patients. *Acta Psychiatrica Scandinavica, 55*(2), 97-101.

Carlson, G. A., Rapport, M. D., Kelly, K. L., & Pataki, C. S. (1992). The effects of methylphenidate and lithium on attention and activity level. *Journal of the American Academy of Child and Adolescent Psychiatry, 31*(2), 262.

Center for Disease Control and Prevention (CDC). (2015, November 9). *Attention-Deficit / Hyperactivity Disorder (ADHD)*. U.S. Department of Health and Human Services. Retrieved from www.cdc.gov/ncbddd/adhd

Dorrego, M. F., Canevaro, L., Kuzis, G., Sabe, L., & Starkstein, S. E. (2002). A randomized, double-blind, crossover study of methylphenidate and lithium in adults with attention-deficit/hyperactivity disorder: Preliminary findings. *Journal of Neuropsychiatry and Clinical Neurosciences, 14*(3), 289-295.

Dykens, E. M., Cassidy, S. B., & DeVries, M. L. (2011). Prader-Willi syndrome. In: S. Goldstein, C. R. Reynolds, S. Goldstein, C. R. Reynolds (eds.), *Handbook of neurodevelopmental and genetic disorders in children*, 2nd ed. New York, NY: Guilford Press. pp. 484-511.

Findling, R. L., Robb, A., McNamara, N. K., Pavuluri, M. N., Kafantaris, V., Scheffer, R., & ... Taylor-Zapata, P. (2015). Lithium in the acute treatment of bipolar I disorder: a double-blind, placebo-controlled study. *Pediatrics, 136*(5), 885-894.

Grohol, J. (2014). *An Introduction to ADHD*. Psych Central. Retrieved from www.psychcentral.com/lib/an-introduction-to-adhd

Gross, H. A., Ebert, M. H., Faden, V. B., Goldberg, S. C., Nee, L. E., & Kaye, W. H. (1981). A double-blind controlled trial of lithium carbonate primary anorexia nervosa. *Journal of Clinical Psychopharmacology, 1*(6), 376-381.

Hsu, L. G. (1984). Treatment of bulimia with lithium. *American Journal of Psychiatry, 141*(10), 1260-1262.

Kotwal, R., Guerdjikova, A., McElroy, S. L., & Keck, P. J. (2006). Lithium augmentation of topiramate for bipolar disorder with comorbid binge eating disorder and obesity. *Human Psychopharmacology: Clinical and Experimental, 21*(7), 425-431.

Masi, G., Milone, A., Manfredi, A., Pari, C., Paziente, A., & Millepiedi, S. (2009). Effectiveness of lithium in children and adolescents with conduct disorder: a retrospective naturalistic study. *CNS Drugs, 23*(1), 59.

McElroy, S., Kotwal, R., & Malhotra, S. (2004). Comorbidity of bipolar disorder and eating disorders: what can the clinician do? *Primary Psychiatry, 11*(10), 36-74.

National Institute of Mental Health (NIMH). (n.d.). "Attention Deficit Hyperactivity Disorder (ADHD)." National Institutes of Health. Retrieved from www.nimh.nih.gov/health/topics/attention-deficit-hyperactivity-disorder-adhd/index.shtml

National Institute of Diabetes and Digestive and Kidney Disorders (NIDDK). (2012). *Binge eating disorders.* National Institutes of Health. Retrieved from www.niddk.nih.gov/health-information/health-topics/weight-control/binge_eating/Pages/binge-eating-disorder.aspx

Forster, J.L., & Gourash, L.M. (2005). *Prader-Willi Syndrome: A Primer for Psychiatrists.* Pittsburgh Partnership. Prader-Willi Syndrome Association USA.

Qiu, M., Ye, Z., Li, Q., Liu, G., Xie, B., & Wang, J. (2011). Changes of Brain Structure and Function in ADHD Children. *Brain Topography, 24*(3-4), 243.

Rubenstein, J. L., Steiner, H., Pratt, J. M., & Koran, L. M. (1991). Anorexia nervosa with bipolar disorder: A case report. *International Journal of Eating Disorders, 10*(2), 221-225.

Verhoeven, W. A., Tuinier, S., & Curfs, L. G. (2003). Prader-Willi syndrome: the psychopathological phenotype in uniparental disomy. *Journal of Medical Genetics, 40*(10), e112.

# Fourteen

## LITHIUM AS A MEDICINE: LYME DISEASE, HEADACHES, GLAUCOMA, AND FIBROMYALGIA

The research continues to accumulate on how important lithium is for healing and regeneration of cells on the nervous system. This simple nutrient has a well-documented ability to restore and balance the complex inner systems of the brain. Throughout this book, we've tapped into the impressive body of literature showing that lithium encourages neuroprotection, repair of neurons, and neurogenesis throughout the lifespan. It is therefore no wonder that over the years, lithium salts have been used in various forms to treat mental health disorders and select neurodegenerative conditions. However, we believe its healing powers have wider-reaching implications.

This chapter focuses on lithium's potential in treating a variety of additional neurological conditions, many of which currently have no cure. Few clinical trials have been undertaken to explore lithium's effect on illnesses outside of mental health; researchers and pharmaceutical companies remain distracted by the production of newer and more profitable drugs. Here we will survey current evidence regarding Lyme disease, cluster headaches, glaucoma, and fibromyalgia, in hopes that this discussion spurs continued investigation into lithium's positive influence on nervous system health.

## Lyme Disease

Lyme disease is caused by the bacterium *Borrelia burgdorferi*, which is transmitted to humans through the bite of an infected tick. Typical symptoms include fever, headache, fatigue, and a characteristic skin rash called erythema migrans. Standard treatment is a few weeks of antibiotics. However, up to 30% of patients receiving a course of antibiotics are not cured with this regimen (Rosner, 2007).

If left unresolved, the infection can spread to joints, the heart, and the nervous system. Lyme neuroborreliosis, also known as neurologic Lyme disease, is the form of Lyme that affects the nervous system. It commonly manifests as mild to moderate cognitive deficits, problems with verbal fluency and short-term memory, and slower processing speed. There have been reports of neuropsychiatric symptoms such as depression, mania, psychosis, and dementia secondary to Lyme disease as well (Fallon et al., 2010). Associated behavioral disorders such as "Lyme rage," violence, and suicidality can also arise.

These troublesome neurological symptoms are believed to result from widespread inflammation in the brain and spinal cord, which occurs as part of the immune system response to the Lyme bacteria. In animal trials, monkeys infected with *Borrelia burgdorferi* showed a dramatic increase in inflammatory markers. There was also a marked rise in apoptosis, or programmed cell death, in spinal cord cells (Ramesh et al., 2013). Likewise, in humans, increased levels of proinflammatory cytokines have been reported in the cerebrospinal fluid of patients with neurologic Lyme disease (Fallon et al., 2010).

There is an abundance of data to suggest lithium has a remediating effect on neurological Lyme patients. Lyme disease infects the central nervous system with toxins, while lithium protects brain cells and preserves brain function. Primarily, lithium helps to reduce brain inflammation, thereby alleviating related symptoms. Lithium does this by increasing anti-inflammatory mediators, as well as supporting antioxidant production to counteract the damaging neurotoxins produced by the Lyme bacteria (Basselin et al., 2010). Lithium has also been found to adjust and balance the rate of apoptosis to protect nerve cells. Bryan Rosner writes in *The Top 10 Lyme Disease Treatments*:

> "So profound are the neuroprotective effects of lithium that numerous Lyme disease sufferers have noticed huge improvements in mood, memory, motivation, aggressive feelings, and other mental functions simply by adding a very small amount of lithium to their supplementation regimens" (Rosner, 2007).

Around the world many Lyme Literate Medical Doctors recommend lithium supplementation as part of a treatment course, although there has yet to be a clinical trial published on the subject. Treatment must also include an antibacterial therapy because Lyme disease begins as a bacterial infection. However, lithium's anti-inflammatory actions could work tangentially to reduce and even eliminate Lyme-related symptoms such as depression, confusion, fatigue, headache, vision problems, and behavioral instability (Rosner, 2007).

## Cluster Headaches

Cluster headache is a neurovascular disorder of which the pathophysiology and etiology are not well understood. As the name suggests, cluster headaches occur in groupings or a course of frequent attacks, during which headaches appear one to three times per day over six to 12 weeks. A single attack can persist anywhere from 15 minutes to three hours, meaning that individuals can experience debilitating pain for hours on end when they are caught in a cluster. Headaches often take place at the same time each day, with most attacks surfacing at night, one to two hours after going to bed. Cluster periods may also arise seasonally, suggesting a circadian component to the disorder. After a cluster period there will be a time of remission, during which the headache attacks stop seemingly spontaneously for months or even years (NINDS, 2013).

Unfortunately, even after a period of remission, cluster headaches can recur quickly and without warning. The most common symptom is excruciating pain, generally located in or around one eye, but it may radiate to other areas of the face, head, neck, or shoulders. This pain is described as sharp, penetrating, or burning. In contrast to those experiencing a migraine, those

# Nutritional Lithium: A Cinderella Story

with cluster headache usually avoid lying down during an attack because this position seems to increase the pain (NINDS, 2013).

The exact cause of cluster headache is unknown. However, since circadian rhythm seems to be involved, abnormalities in the hypothalamus likely play a role. Our biological clock is located in the hypothalamus, which lies deep in the center of the brain. Additionally, imaging studies have discovered increased activity in the hypothalamus during a bout of cluster headaches.

The main prophylactic therapies for both episodic and chronic cluster headaches are verapamil, an anti-hypertensive, and lithium (Becker, 2013). The efficacy of lithium for headaches was first discovered and officially tested in the 1970's. Dr. Nieper treated a group of 44 patients aged 15-74 who suffered from constant headaches, migraines, and hemicranias with low-dose lithium in the form of lithium orotate. All were dissatisfied with the results of previous treatments (including ergotamine, caffeine, lithium citrate, lithium carbonate). For some patients, previous therapy had lessened the severity of headaches, but failed to prevent them altogether. Other patients reported therapies they tried in the past were totally ineffective or caused unpleasant side effects. Each week Nieper administered 5-6 capsules of 150 mg lithium orotate. After lithium orotate therapy, sensations that usually accompany migraine attacks, such as flicker scotoma, disappeared in all patients. Thirty-nine patients reported lithium to be thoroughly effective. The five patients who saw no improvement may have suffered from headaches of a structural, rather than neurochemical, origin (Nieper, 1973).

In another experiment, researchers administered slow release lithium tablets (6 mEq) to five male patients ages 26 to 57 with cluster headache, three of whom had chronic symptoms. For the three suffering from chronic headaches, lithium resulted in an immediate, partial remission of the headaches. The headaches increased in intensity and frequency when lithium was withdrawn and improved again when the mineral was re-administered. Placebo had no effect. In the two patients with periodic symptoms, lithium also appeared to be efficacious. Even though the dose of lithium was significantly higher than the supplemental levels evaluated in Dr. Nieper's original study, no serious side effects were observed over the duration of the study or in follow-up periods (Ekbom, 1977).

## Lithium as a Medicine: Lyme Disease, Headaches, Glaucoma,...

In another study published around the same time, pharmaceutical lithium also proved useful for treating cluster headaches. Thirty-two patients were treated with lithium carbonate 300-600 mg a day during the first week followed by 600-900 mg by the fourth week. Lithium led to dramatic relief during the first week, and patients remained almost symptom free for the duration of this study. Moderately long-term therapy did not lead to lithium tolerance, and even lower lithium maintenance doses provided continued improvement after the twelfth week. Three patients dropped out early in the study due to "lithium headache", a side effect of high-dose lithium resulting in severe throbbing occipital pain. When lithium was stopped, there was complete relief from "lithium headache" (Kudrow, 1977). Lower doses were not explored in this particular study, but may have proven useful for those responding poorly to highly concentrated doses of the mineral.

Studies conducted more recently also support the use of lithium in the treatment of headaches. The effect of lithium was evaluated in a sample of 26 patients diagnosed with episodic cluster headache. Dosage of lithium varied from 450 to 1,050 mg/day. Twenty patients (77%) were responders and six (23%) were classified as nonresponders. Responders were defined as patients showing at least a 50% reduction in attack frequency. Fifteen of the 20 responders showed significant clinical improvement by the end of the first week, and the remaining five improved during the second week. Adverse drug reactions were reported in 15% of study participants, primarily when high doses were given for extended periods of time. The study authors therefore recommended lithium as an episodic treatment, and warned that pharmaceutical doses should only be used over the long term when other medications prove ineffective or potentially harmful (Stochino et al., 2012). Again, researchers neglected to question whether lowering the dose would mediate ill effects while sustaining therapeutic benefits. Future research should work towards establishing this threshold.

It remains unclear as exactly how lithium works to produce both rapid and lasting relief from cluster headaches. As discussed previously, cluster headaches are characterized by a cyclic nature and hormonal alterations, which indicate involvement of the hypothalamus in pathogenesis. One possible mechanism of action of lithium is thus its effect on the serotonin level in the hypothalamus. One study has linked headache relief with lithium's effect on platelet serotonin and histamine levels. It has also been proposed that lithium alleviates headache symptoms by shifting opiate receptor affinity. Two further studies reported that the immediate action of lithium in treating cluster headache is related to its effect on REM sleep (Abdel-Maksoud et al., 2009). Taken altogether, the collective message from this research is that lithium, at a range of doses, provides neurological support to relieve cluster headache symptoms on an acute and prophylactic basis.

## Glaucoma

Glaucoma is a progressive eye condition that damages the optic nerve—a group of nerve fibers that transmit images to the brain. Impairments result from a buildup of pressure inside the eye, called intraocular pressure, which strains and degrades the optic nerve over time. Without treatment, glaucoma can cause total permanent blindness within a few years. However, most people with glaucoma will not go blind if they follow their treatment plan and have regular eye exams (AOA, 2015).

Patients with glaucoma typically have few or no symptoms. The first sign is often loss of peripheral vision. If intraocular pressure rises to severe levels, sudden eye pain, headache, blurred vision, or the appearance of halos around lights may occur. Glaucoma most often occurs gradually in adults over the age of 40. In African-Americans, glaucoma presents more frequently, at an earlier age and with greater loss of vision. There is additional risk of glaucoma with a family history of the disease, poor vision, or diabetes. These statistics suggests that both genetic and lifestyle factors contribute to glaucoma etiology (AOA, 2015).

Interest in the use of lithium for glaucoma came from Dr. Nieper's early studies using low-dose lithium for headache sufferers. Study participants suffering from the visual abnormalities associated with migraines, including increased intraocular pressure and myopia (nearsightedness), seemed to benefit greatly from supplemental levels of the mineral (Nieper, 1973). Dr. Nieper predicted that lithium had a slight dehydrating effect on the eye, which resulted in improved vision and a reduction of intraocular pressure.

In spite of these exciting findings, a follow-up study didn't appear until years later. In 2014, researchers using a glaucoma rat model found that lithium chloride reduced intraocular pressure by about 22% in a six-week period (Sun et al., 2014). Their explanation for lithium's glaucoma-fighting effects was far more complex than Nieper's original dehydration hypothesis, however. Using advanced technology these researchers were able to see that lithium reduced intraocular pressure by stimulating cell membrane proteins that are activated under stress to protect and promote nerve cell survival. In particular, lithium triggered the release of compounds known to slow the progression of optic neuropathy and promote the regeneration of crushed retinal cell axons (Sun et al., 2014). Therefore, lithium may enhance neuroprotection and neurogenesis in optic nerve cells, making it an encouraging therapy for glaucoma patients.

## Fibromyalgia

Fibromyalgia is a disorder characterized by widespread musculoskeletal pain, accompanied by fatigue and issues with sleep, memory, and mood. It is the second most common musculoskeletal condition diagnosed today, with almost 12 million sufferers in the United States alone. Researchers believe that fibromyalgia is the result of neurological abnormalities, including altered neurotransmitter levels and a hyper-sensitization of pain receptors in the brain.

The primary symptom of fibromyalgia is widespread pain felt over the entire body. The pain can be deep, sharp, dull, throbbing, or aching, and is felt in the muscles, tendons, and ligaments around the joints. In addition to generalized muscle soreness and body aches, people with fibromyalgia may have painful localized areas of tenderness around their joints, called tender points, which hurt when pressed with a finger. Depression is also a major symptom; up to half of all people with fibromyalgia have depression or an anxiety disorder when they are diagnosed (Williamson, 2009).

Initial treatment is usually an antidepressant which helps relieve pain, fatigue, and problems with mood and sleep. Tricyclic antidepressants have been used for many years to treat fibromyalgia. These medications work by raising the levels of serotonin and norepinephrine in the brain. Those suffering from chronic pain frequently have diminished levels of these calming neurotransmitters. Treatment with tricyclics is often very effective, but multiple side effects such as drowsiness, dizziness, dry mouth, dry eyes, and constipation can make the medications hard to tolerate (Williamson, 2009).

Although robust trials are lacking, lithium may provide relief from fibromyalgia symptoms. Lithium carbonate and tricyclic antidepressants have been previously used together successfully. Lithium may augment the antidepressant effect of tricyclic antidepressants in resistant unipolar depression, as discussed in an earlier chapter. Furthermore, one type of tricyclic antidepressant, amitriptyline, has been effectively used in conjunction with lithium for treating painful shoulder syndrome. Since those with fibromyalgia commonly present with depression and painful shoulder syndrome, lithium may be a useful adjunct to tricyclic antidepressants therapy for fibromyalgia (Tyber, 1990).

In 1990, Dr. Tyber reported on three cases of fibromyalgia that were resistant to tricyclic antidepressants therapy. The patients improved greatly after the addition of lithium. In all three women, lithium reduced pain and stiffness. Laboratory tests showed no evidence of lithium toxicity within the thyroid or the kidney (Tyber, 1990). Two anesthesiologists, Toinette Fontrier and John Lewis, have been studying fibromyalgia for years. Dr. Fontrier, who has been disabled by fibromyalgia herself, explains that after excess activity, her pain can become debilitating, affecting all aspects of her life and preventing sleep. Her pain is not responsive to opioids, NSAIDs, or gabapentin. However, 300 mg of lithium carbonate will decrease her pain by 70–80% within 40 minutes. The effect lasts 4-5 hours. The benefit of lithium is dramatic and reproducible (Fontrier, 2004).

Fontrier and Lewis believe fibromyalgia may be related to a calcium-parathyroid axis dysfunction (Fontrier, 2004). They propose that the results seen in Tyber's three case studies may be related to the fact that lithium can raise serum levels of parathyroid hormone (Lewis & Fontrier, 2003). Further study is needed to define exactly how lithium works to assuage the pain and mood symptoms seen in fibromyalgia.

## Achieving Neurological Health with Lithium
Lithium has been studied and continually examined under the lens of skeptics in psychiatry. After years of study, the mineral has been shown to have diverse effects, including its abilities to balance neurotransmitter levels, decrease inflammation in the brain, and stimulate nerve cell growth to stabilize mood. Lithium is a life-saving treatment for many mental health patients, but this brain-saving nutrient has clinical implications for the treatment and prevention of several neurodegenerative conditions as well.

The neuroprotective, neuroreparative and neurogenerative features of lithium could be harnessed for the treatment of many other neurobiological conditions. A limited but heartening group of studies exists to show that lithium may help to alleviate neuropsychiatric symptoms in Lyme disease, ease pain in cluster headache sufferers, stop the progression of glaucoma, and restore a sense of normalcy in the lives of patients with fibromyalgia. These data support the notion that lithium, at nutritional and pharmacological doses, can result in clinical improvement in a variety of nervous system conditions. Further research should investigate lithium's precise role in the nervous system and determine optimal intake for neurological health.

# Nutritional Lithium: A Cinderella Story

## CHAPTER 14 | References

Abdel-Maksoud, M. B., Nasr, A., & Abdul-Aziz, A. (2009). Lithium treatment in cluster headache, review of literature. *European Journal of Psychiatry, 23*(1), 53-60.

Adityanjee. (1995). Modification of clozapine-induced leukopenia and neutropenia with lithium carbonate. *American Journal of Psychiatry, 152*(4), 648-9.

American Optometric Association (AOA). (2015). *Glaucoma.* Retrieved from www.aoa.org/patients-and-public/eye-and-vision-problems/glossary-of-eye-and-vision-conditions/glaucoma

Ballin, A., Lehman, D., Sirota, P., Litvinjuk, U., & Meytes, D. (1998). Increased number of peripheral blood CD34+ cells in lithium-treated patients. *British Journal of Haematology, 100*(1), 219-221.

Basselin, M., Kim, H., Chen, M., Ma, K., Rapoport, S. I., Murphy, R. C., & Farias, S. E. (2010). Lithium modifies brain arachidonic and docosahexaenoic metabolism in rat lipopolysaccharide model of neuroinflammation. *Journal of Lipid Research, 51*(5), 1049-1056.

Becker, W. J. (2013). Cluster Headache: Conventional Pharmacological Management. *Headache: The Journal of Head & Face Pain, 53*(7), 1191-1196.

Bender, S., Linka, T., Wolstein, J., Gehendges, S., Paulus, H., Schall, U., & Gastpar, M. (2004). Safety and efficacy of combined clozapine-lithium pharmacotherapy. *International Journal of Neuropsychopharmacology, 7*(1), 59-63.

Brunoni, A. R., Kobuti Ferreira, L. R., Gallucci-Neto, J., Elkis, H., Velloso, E. R., & Vinicius Zanetti, M. (2008). Lithium as a treatment of clozapine-induced neutropenia: a case report. *Progress in Neuro-Psychopharmacology & Biological Psychiatry, 32*(8), 2006-2007.

Ekbom, K. (1977). Lithium in the Treatment of Chronic Cluster Headache. *Headache: The Journal of Head & Face Pain, 17*(1), 39.

Fallon, B. A., Levin, E. S., Schweitzer, P. J., & Hardesty, D. (2010). Inflammation and central nervous system Lyme disease. *Inflammation in Neuropsychiatric Disease, 37*(3), 534-541.

Fontrier, T. (2004). Lithium for fibromyalgia. *Anesthesia and Analgesia, 98*(5), 1505.

Kessler, L., Palla, J., Baru, J. S., Onyenwenyi, C., George, A. M., & Lucas, B. P. (2014). Lithium as an adjunct to radioactive iodine for the treatment of hyperthyroidism: a systematic review and meta-analysis. *Endocrine Practice: Official Journal of the American College of Endocrinology and the American Association of Clinical Endocrinologists, 20*(7), 737-745.

Kudrow, L. (1977). Lithium Prophylaxis for Chronic Cluster Headache. *Headache: The Journal of Head & Face Pain, 17*(1), 15.

Lewis, J., & Fontrier, T. (2003). Lithium and fibromyalgia. *Journal of Musculoskeletal Pain, 11*(1), 69-70.

Lingudu, B., Bongi, V., Ayyagari, M., & Venkata, S. (2014). Impact of lithium on radioactive iodine therapy for hyperthyroidism. *Indian Journal of Endocrinology And Metabolism, 18*(5), 669-75.

National Institute of Neurological Disorders and Stroke (NINDS). (2013). *Headache: Hope through Research.* National Institutes of Health. Retrieved from www.ninds.nih.gov/disorders/headache/detail_headache.htm

Nieper, H. A. (1973). The clinical applications of lithium orotate. A two years study. *Agressologie, 14*(6), 407-411.

Ramesh, G., Santana-Gould, L., Inglis, F. M., et al. (2013). The Lyme disease spirochete Borrelia burgdorferi induces inflammation and apoptosis in cells from dorsal root ganglia. *Journal of Neuroinflammation, 10*, 88.

Reid, J., & Wheeler, S. (2005). Hyperthyroidism: diagnosis and treatment. *American Family Physician, 72*(4), 623-569.

Rosner, B. (2007). *The Top 10 Lyme Disease Treatments: Defeat Lyme Disease with the Best of Conventional and Alternative Medicine.* South Lake Tahoe, CA: BioMed Publishing Group.

Stein, R. S., Beaman, C., Ali, M. Y., Hansen, R., Jenkins, D. D., & Jume'an, H. G. (1977). Lithium carbonate attenuation of chemotherapy-induced neutropenia. *New England Journal of Medicine, 297*(8), 430-431.

Stochino, M. E., Deidda, A., Asuni, C., Cherchi, A., Manchia, M., & Del Zompo, M. (2012). Evaluation of Lithium Response in Episodic Cluster

Headache: A Retrospective Case Series. *Headache: The Journal of Head & Face Pain, 52*(7), 1171-1175.

Sun, X., Lu, H., Chen, Y., Fan, X., & Tong, B. (2014). Effect of lithium chloride on endoplasmic reticulum stress-related PERK/ROCK signaling in a rat model of glaucoma. *Die Pharmazie, 69*(12), 889-893.

Tyber, M. A. (1990). Lithium carbonate augmentation therapy in fibromyalgia. *Canadian Medical Association Journal, 143*(9), 902.

U.S. Food and Drug Administration. (2015). *FDA Drug Safety Communication: FDA modifies monitoring for neutropenia associated with schizophrenia medicine clozapine; approves new shared REMS program for all clozapine medicines.* Retrieved from www.fda.gov/Drugs/DrugSafety/ucm461853.htm

Williamson, M. (2009). *Fibromyalgia: A comprehensive approach: What you can do about chronic pain and fatigue.* New York, NY: Walker Publishing Company.

Zhuang, J., Li, F., Liu, X., et al. (2009). Lithium chloride protects retinal neurocytes from nutrient deprivation by promoting DNA non-homologous end-joining. *Biochemical and Biophysical Research Communications, 380,* 650-654.

# Fifteen

## THE ROLE OF LITHIUM IN INTEGRATIVE PSYCHIATRY

I wrote this book to share one of the most exciting and effective medical interventions I have found in over 25 years of practice. It would be impossible for me to overstate the benefits I have seen from using lithium in my clinical practice.

A deficiency in lithium can underlie a wide array of psychiatric and neurological symptoms. Simply, the body needs lithium to ensure healthy metabolism in the brain. Although lithium has long been part of the pharmacologist's armamentarium for treating bipolar disorder, my clinical experience and growing research studies have also shown that lithium is a fundamental part of nutritional medicine and therefore of integrative psychiatry. In addition to the several medical and psychiatric conditions discussed in this book, patients who have struggled with obsessive-compulsive disorder (OCD), post-traumatic stress disorder (PTSD), and anxiety disorders have also responded well to nutritional lithium. Regardless of psychiatric diagnosis, I have observed countless patients benefit from nutritional lithium.

## Orthomolecular Psychiatry

The notion that mental health treatment can be improved with nutritional substances is not new. In the 1960's, Nobel Laureate Linus Pauling encouraged physicians to help restore patients to health through treatment with natural substances (Pauling, 1968). He and Abram Hoffer developed a discipline they called *orthomolecular medicine*. Orthomolecular medicine is based on an understanding of the key role of nutrients in health and disease. They recognized that chemicals entering the body need to go through various enzymatic transformations on the way to producing neurotransmitters. To optimize the speed and efficiency of metabolism, the body needs cofactors, or nutrients. These nutrients are the precursors to essential neurotransmitters that sustain brain health.

An important tenet of orthomolecular psychiatry is awareness of biochemical individuality: each of us is unique with a biochemical signature as distinctive as our fingerprints (Williams, 1998). Conversely, the unspoken basis of traditional psychiatry is sameness. Individuals are grouped into symptom-based disorder categories delineated by the *Diagnostic and Statistical Manual of Mental Disorders (DSM)* even though each of us is a distinct individual with a unique biochemical profile. Orthomolecular psychiatry emphasizes that the challenges of improving mental health lie in identifying an individual's nutrient deficiencies and correcting them.

The past century has witnessed considerable research on the importance of various nutrients for brain cells and deficiencies of those nutrients as the basis of brain dysfunction in individual patients. Yet important findings from scientific research have not been incorporated into most medical school training programs. As a medical student, I was fascinated by nutrition and the possibility that nutritional interventions could prevent and treat disease. But nutrition had no part in the existing curriculum. I completed my medical training as a psychopharmacologist, meaning that I was trained to treat psychiatric problems by prescribing medications. Eventually, I realized that many psychiatric illnesses are not primarily psychiatric problems, but biological ones. I saw that correcting nutritional imbalances and ensuring that my patients consumed adequate amounts of vitamins, minerals, amino acids, and fatty acids were critical in restoring brain health and laying the foundation for a long-lasting recovery. Moreover, adequate nutrition supports psychotherapy and mind-body practices including yoga, and even helps medication work more effectively.

## The Role of Lithium in Integrative Psychiatry

That was three decades ago. Still today, nutrition is often neglected or considered in the domain of "alternative" medicine. Many psychiatrists seem to believe they must be entrenched in one camp or the other; they must either practice traditional Western medicine and focus on dispensing prescriptions, or be labeled as "alternative" and abandon what they have learned about pharmacological treatment. As a practitioner of integrative medicine, I believe our patients deserve access to all interventions to support and improve mental health.

The link between nutrition and psychological symptoms has been recorded for centuries. Pellagra is an example of how a deficiency in a single nutrient, vitamin B3 (niacin), can have profound implications for brain function and produce identical symptoms to schizophrenia. In 1944, Ancel Keys, a physiology professor at the University of Minnesota, launched a landmark study of the effects of starvation on the body (Keys et al., 1950). Men who had been Conscientious Objectors during World War II were enlisted in the Minnesota Starvation Experiment. Under conditions that combined a severely restricted caloric intake and intense exercise, the men gradually exhibited typical psychological characteristics of anorexia, depression, OCD, anxiety, irritability, and delusional thinking. They had been psychologically healthy before the study; they developed psychological symptoms because their bodies had been deprived of nutrients.

There is extensive scientific literature describing the relationship between nutritional deficiencies and brain health. Nearly 20 years ago, psychiatrist Joseph Hibbeln MD found that a group of prisoners who were given omega 3 fatty acid supplements committed strikingly fewer aggressive acts than a placebo group (Hibbeln et al., 1996). Hibbeln and his colleagues continued to examine the effectiveness of this supplement in later studies and found that study participants supplemented with omega-3 fatty acids had significantly greater improvements in scores for depression and reductions in markers for suicidal behavior (Hibbeln et al., 2006; Hallahan et al., 2007). In 2015, Australian researchers also found that volunteer inmates who had extremely low levels of omega-3 fatty acids also displayed the worst levels of aggression and impulsivity (Meyer et al., 2015). The implications present a promising opportunity: nutritional interventions can diminish the anger and agitation that drive violent behavior.

An integrative approach to psychiatric treatment derives in part from insights of orthomolecular psychiatry and relies significantly on nutritional therapies. It also builds on contributions of recent research. New information from the fields of genetics, neurobiology, and neuroimaging support the realization that psychiatric disorders are based in biology. New research confirms that without essential nutrients, the body cannot build cells, grow normally, or heal properly (Kaplan et al., 2015). Nearly all cellular processes, from gene expression to protein synthesis, are affected by diet. The new field of nutrigenomics focuses on using nutritional strategies to switch off genes that make people susceptible to mental disorders, and encouraging a nutritious diet that sets the stage for a helpful rather than a harmful epigenome (Sarris et al., 2015).

Nutrition is not only an important part of treatment for mental disorders; it has a significant role to play in prevention as well. New research confirms the preventive benefits of nutritional substances. For example, long-chain omega 3 polyunsaturated fatty acids (PUFAs) are necessary for neural development and function, and a lack of these fatty acids is implicated in a number of mental health conditions, including schizophrenia (Amminger et al., 2010). Recent research has shown that adolescents with subthreshold schizophrenia who take PUFA supplements in the form of low-dose fish oil are significantly less likely to develop psychosis than those who do not take supplements (Amminger et al., 2015). The differences persist at least 6 years after the initial dose. For years, I have alerted patients and their parents about vitamin, mineral, and fatty acid deficiencies as precursors to eating disorders. Although seldom featured in either the professional or lay press, these studies that confirm my clinical observations definitively establish the power of nutrition as a model for prevention (Greenblatt, 2011).

And why has the wisdom that emerges so clearly from these studies been so difficult for our field to integrate? One possible explanation for the reluctance of the medical community to recognize the benefits of nutritional therapies is a phenomenon called the *tomato effect*. The tomato effect, identified by Dr. James Goodwin in 1984, occurs when an efficacious treatment for a certain disease is ignored or rejected because it does not make sense in light of accepted theories of disease mechanism and drug action. The rejection of potentially useful treatment because everyone knows it won't work is named for American's stubborn belief—from the 16$^{th}$ to 19$^{th}$ centuries—that tomatoes were poisonous. Despite mounting evidence, most physicians discount treatment strategies that do not fit into the framework of health and disease that they studied (Goodwin, 1984).

## Lithium as Nutritional Intervention

Within my integrative approach to treating brain health, I have found lithium the single most important nutrient for the treatment and prevention of psychiatric disorders. Lithium is a significant cofactor in nearly every enzymatic function in every pathway of the brain. Lithium stimulates neurogenesis. One brain region involved with rebirth and regulation of neuron cells is the hippocampus, the gray structure in the center of the brain responsible for learning, memory, mood, and emotion. Lithium is associated with increases in size of the hippocampus. Hippocampal neurons are important for learning and memory. The ability of the brain to produce new neurons may protect against depression, anxiety, and other mental health issues. Nothing on the planet—natural or synthetic—appears to support neurogenesis better than lithium.

Moreover, studies in epigenetics have shown that lithium can treat and prevent psychiatric illness in predisposed individuals by switching on processes that foster brain health while switching off processes that deteriorate brain cells. Lithium works on both histone modification and changes in DNA methylation and influences the expression of more than 50 genes.

An area of important research focuses on identifying ways to promote the survival of neurons as synapses degrade with age, stress, and environmental stressors over time. One of the fascinating properties of lithium is that it is able to stimulate the release of proteins that regulate the growth and survival of neurons, such as brain-derived neurotrophic factor (BDNF). BDNF is the most prevalent growth factor in the central nervous system, and protects the brain by increasing levels of other neurotrophic factors.

As a medicine, lithium is the gold standard for treating bipolar disorder. It is also effective in treating other psychiatric illnesses, including recurrent depression, suicidal tendencies, substance abuse, and ADHD. Lithium has shown benefits in treating patients with neurological disorders such as Parkinson's disease and Alzheimer's disease. Research also shows that lithium can help alleviate symptoms of eating disorders, headaches, glaucoma, and anemia. Promising new research shows lithium as an effective adjuvant therapy for treating the neurological changes in Lyme disease and cognitive decline that result from chemotherapy, as well as ameliorating symptoms of amyotrophic lateral sclerosis (ALS), PTSD, and traumatic brain injuries (Zanni et al., 2015).

Clinical use of lithium is also associated with reduced cancer incidence in psychiatric patients. In an early report, cancer incidence was significantly lower in the group of 609 psychiatric patients treated with lithium when compared with 2,396 controls. Other studies have also found that lithium treatment suppressed tumor growth in human cancer cells (Zhu et al., 2011).

In the presence of genetic polymorphisms, metabolic changes (pregnancy, post-partum, or aging), or disease states (diabetes, cancer), individuals possess unique nutritional needs. Smokers have higher nutritional requirements for vitamin C due to increased oxidative damage. Alcoholics need thiamine above the Recommended Daily Intake requirement to prevent Wernicke's encephalopathy. The mutation found in the methylenetetrahydrofolate reductase (MTHFR) gene is caused by a common single nucleotide polymorphism that is associated with increased incidence of depression (Kelly et al., 2004). The genetic polymorphism can be circumvented by the addition of L-methylfolate supplementation, which can yield improved treatment outcomes for depressed patients.

The core concepts of integrative medicine and biochemical individuality are embedded in the understanding that optimal doses of any nutrient will vary between individuals (Williams, 1998). Lithium is an essential nutrient without a formally named deficiency syndrome defined by our current models. Regardless, the available scientific literature demonstrates the overwhelming importance of lithium in brain health and mental illness. For some individuals, nutritional lithium may be required in higher doses than it can be obtained through dietary intake alone.

The story of lithium is a true Cinderella story. Lithium is a common and simple element, and was among one of the first three elements produced within minutes after the Big Bang that created this universe (Peebles, 1991). Its benefits have not been heralded, as the fanfare associated with lucrative pharmaceuticals eclipses its simplicity. When newer treatments appear on the market, lithium is treated like Cinderella, often ignored and forgotten.

But like Cinderella, lithium shows great promise. Its nature is deceptive because it holds the power to transform lives. From stardust to consciousness, lithium has unique properties as a mineral, a medicine, and a miracle.

## CHAPTER 15 | References

Amminger, G. P., Schafer, M. R., Papageorgiou, K., Klier, C. M., Cotton, S. M., Harrigan, S. M., & ... Berger, G. E. (2010). Long-chain omega-3 fatty acids for indicated prevention of psychotic disorders: a randomized, placebo-controlled trial. *Archives of General Psychiatry, 67*(2), 146.

Amminger, G. P., Schäfer, M. R., Schlögelhofer, M., Klier, C. M., & McGorry, P. D. (2015). Longer-term outcome in the prevention of psychotic disorders by the Vienna omega-3 study. *Nature Communications, 6,* 7934.

Goodwin, J. S., & Goodwin, J. M. (1984). The tomato effect. Rejection of highly efficacious therapies. *JAMA, 251*(18), 2387-2390.

Greenblatt, J. M. (2010). *Answers to anorexia: A breakthrough nutritional treatment that is saving lives,* North Branch, MN: Sunrise River Press.

Hallahan, B., Hibbeln, J.R., Davis, J. M., & Garland, M.R. (2007). Omega-3 fatty acid supplementation in patients with recurrent self-harm. *British Journal of Psychiatry, 190*(2), 118-122.

Hibbeln, J. R., Umhau, J. C., George, D. T., & Salem, N. J. (1997). Do plasma polyunsaturates predict hostility and depression? *World Review of Nutrition and Dietetics, 82,* 175-186.

Hibbeln, J.R., Ferguson, T.A., & Blasbalg, T.L. (2006). Omega-3 fatty acid deficiencies in neurodevelopment, aggression, and autonomic dysregulation: opportunities for intervention. *International Review of Psychiatry, 18*(2), 107-118.

Kalm, L. M., & Semba, R. D. (2005). They starved so that others be better fed: remembering Ancel Keys and the Minnesota Experiment. *Journal of Nutrition, 135*(6), 1347.

Kaplan, B.J., Rucklidge, J.J., Romijn, A., & McLeod, K. (2015). The emerging field of nutritional mental health: inflammation, the microbiome, oxidative stress, and mitochondrial function. *Clinical Psychological Science, 3*(6), 964-980.

Keys, A., Brožek, J., Henschel, A., Mickelsen, O., & Taylor, H. L. (1950). *The biology of human starvation. (2 vols).* St. Paul, MN: University of Minnesota Press.

Kelly, C. B., McDonnell, A. P., Johnston, T. G., Mulholland, C., Cooper, S. J., McMaster, D., & ... Whitehead, A. S. (2004). The MTHFR C677T polymorphism is associated with depressive episodes in patients from Northern Ireland. *Journal of Psychopharmacology, 18*(4), 567-571.

Meyer, B. J., Byrne, M. K., Collier, C., Parletta, N., Crawford, D., Winberg, P. C., & ... Grant, L. (2015). Baseline omega-3 index correlates with aggressive and attention deficit disorder behaviors in adult prisoners. *PLoS One, 10*(3), e0120220.

Mischley, L. (2012). Lithium deficiency in Parkinson's disease. University of Washington MPH thesis. Unpublished.

Pauling, L. (1968). Orthomolecular psychiatry. *Science, 160*(3825), 265-271.

Peebles, P.J., Schramm, D.N., Turner, E.I., & Kron, R.G. (1991). The case for the relativistic hot Big Bang cosmology. *Nature, 352,* 769-776.

Sarris, J., Logan, A. C., Akbaraly, T. N., Amminger, G. P., Balanzá-Martínez, V., Freeman, M. P., & ... Jacka, F. N. (2015). Nutritional medicine as mainstream in psychiatry. *The Lancet. Psychiatry, 2*(3), 271-274.

Williams, R. (1998). *Biochemical Individuality.* New York, NY: McGraw-Hill Education.

Zanni, G., Di Martino, E., Omelyanenko, A., Andäng, M., Delle, U., Elmroth, K., & Blomgren, K. (2015). Lithium increases proliferation of hippocampal neural stem/progenitor cells and rescues irradiation-induced cell cycle arrest in vitro. *Oncotarget, 6*(35), 37083-37097.

Zhu, Q., Yang, J., Han, S., Liu, J., Holzbeierlein, J., Thrasher, J. B., & Li, B. (2011). Suppression of glycogen synthase kinase 3 activity reduces tumor growth of prostate cancer in vivo. *The Prostate, 71*(8), 835-845.

# Author Bios

## James M. Greenblatt, MD

James M. Greenblatt, MD currently serves as the Chief Medical Officer at Walden Behavioral Care in Waltham, MA and serves as an Assistant Clinical Professor of Psychiatry at Tufts University School of Medicine and recently has been appointment to Dartmouth Faculty as a Clinical Assistant Professor of Psychiatry. After receiving his medical degree and completing his psychiatry residency at George Washington University, Dr. Greenblatt went on to complete a fellowship in child and adolescent psychiatry at Johns Hopkins Medical School. Dr. Greenblatt's knowledge in the areas of biology, genetics, psychology, and nutrition as they interact in the treatment of mental illness has led to his editing of a professional text on depression as well as published books for the public and professional audience. His books include *The Breakthrough Depression Solution*, *Answers to Binge Eating*, *Answers to Anorexia*, and *Integrative Therapies for Depression*.

## Kayla Grossmann, RN

Kayla Grossmann, RN, works as a nurse advocate and educator specializing in integrative health research and practice. She supports several large organizations in the field by contributing to ongoing outreach initiatives and clinical programming. Kayla serves as a health consultant and lead content creator for the Radiant Life Company and maintains an active integrative yoga practice in Southern New Hampshire.

# Appendix

## Clinical Case Histories

This book reviewed a vast collection of scientific literature in the areas of medicine, nutrition, biochemistry, psychiatry, and neurology and its relation to lithium. My positive clinical experience with nutritional lithium has been repeated with hundreds of patients. Here are a few examples.

### JENNIFER

I first met Jennifer almost 10 years ago when she was 17 years old. Prior to meeting with me, she had spent the last three years in and out of psychiatric hospitals for classic symptoms characteristic of bipolar disorder. She experienced intense periods of mania with hyper-religiosity, alternating with severe depression with multiple suicide attempts. When she wasn't admitted in psychiatric hospitals, she was meeting with experts across the country in hopes of finding relief from her bipolar disorder.

While in the hospital, she was prescribed multiple medications which provided modest relief, but the side effects were intolerable. She became extremely agitated on antipsychotic medications. When she started on 300 mg of prescription lithium, she reported feeling "flat" and over-sedated, and she suffered from brain fog so severe she was unable to function.

From my clinical assessment which includes a thorough family history, I learned that her maternal grandmother also suffers from bipolar disorder. On her Hair Tissue Mineral Analysis, she had no detectable lithium present. I

## Appendix

recommended a sub-therapeutic dose of lithium, but due to her prior experience with prescription lithium, both Jennifer and her parents were reluctant, so we started by establishing a program for nutritional support.

Based on her nutritional laboratory testing, she began supplemental magnesium, zinc, vitamin D, and vitamin B12. After three months of nutritional support, her family observed modest improvement in her mood and symptoms and agreed to try low-dose lithium orotate. I started off at 5 mg and titrated up to 10 mg twice daily, for a total dose of 20 mg per day. The recovery process was gradual but steady throughout the first year on nutritional lithium. She was not hospitalized, and reported that her mood cycling drastically improved.

Jennifer was able to graduate high school and complete her college studies, and has remained free from psychiatric hospitalizations for the last decade. At present, she continues to take 10 mg of nutritional lithium and reports doing well. She does her regular blood tests and has never had side effects.

### CARL

Carl, a 40-year-old male and a father of three children, struggled with a long history of obsessive-compulsive disorder (OCD). His intrusive thoughts interfered with his performance at work, and the relationships with his loved ones also suffered. He was limited in his ability to spend adequate time with his children due to his intrusive thoughts.

Since the age of 20, he has tried every class of psychotropic medications, including antidepressants, antipsychotics, and mood stabilizers. After nearly two decades of trial and error with various medication combinations and dosages, he found the most relief on a combination of Zoloft 200 mg and Seroquel 25 mg twice daily, but the intrusive thoughts would still interfere with his activities of daily living.

When we reviewed his family history, he shared that his parents both suffered from substance abuse disorders. His Hair Tissue Mineral Analysis also revealed non-detectable lithium. Without changing his medications, I added 5 mg of lithium orotate. Within a few weeks, he reported an improvement in sleep and a decrease in his OCD symptoms.

# Nutritional Lithium: A Cinderella Story

Over the next couple of months, his anxiety diminished, and the frequency of his OCD thoughts lessened, and he was able to return to work and resume activities without disruptions. Over the course of the year, he continued to report progress and stated that he was able to spend more time with his children and improve his relationship that was thought to be impossible before. He was appreciative and relieved that he could finally be a better father toward his children. He continues to take his current medications with nutritional lithium.

## SAM

Sam, an 8-year-old boy, struggled with severe behavioral problems. His parents were often brought in for parent and teacher conferences. where teachers remarked that Samuel was precocious and intelligent, but also debilitated by his inability to focus. He was also easily agitated, aggressive toward other children, and disruptive in the classroom. Samuel's parents brought him for evaluations by several experts who diagnosed him with attention-deficit hyperactivity disorder (ADHD). Samuel was started on stimulant medications that were not helpful, and only caused him to become more agitated. He tried multiple stimulants, and experienced side effects with all of them.

When we completed the nutritional testing, his Hair Tissue Mineral Analysis showed non-detectable lithium. I started Sam on low-dose lithium, and his parents and school teachers noticed an improvement in his behavior within two weeks. Over the course of the next two months, Sam was less disruptive in class and able to participate in activities with his peers, and he lost interest in bullying other children. He has remained on nutritional lithium for two years without behavioral difficulties at school.

## BRIAN

Brian was a middle-aged male who presented for a consultation to address his aggression and irritability. I had no trouble imagining these problems after I was unavoidably 15 minutes behind for our scheduled appointment. He berated me for most of my session, and I later discovered that he was verbally abusive toward my staff. From my meeting with Brian, I learned that he

# Appendix

suffered from depression and was taking an antidepressant medication, but his constant irritability was unresolved. His wife, who appeared later with him to the appointment, reported that his road rage had escalated to such an intensity that he would get out of his car to yell at other drivers.

Without changing his medications, I recommended a low dose of lithium to alleviate his irritability. After a few weeks, he reported feeling less agitated, and both he and his wife stated in a follow-up appointment after eight weeks that his boiling road rage had subsided to nothing more than mild frustration.

## PATRICIA

With the case of Patricia, all of the assessment strategies—clinical history, family history, and results from the Hair Tissue Mineral Analysis—proved to be instrumental in providing relief from her symptoms. As a 43-year-old therapist, Patricia had been diagnosed with depression at the age of 18 and struggled with alcohol abuse throughout her young adulthood. Patricia had been taking an antidepressant medication since the age of 18, and was working hard to maintain her sobriety for the last 10 years. Patricia also shared that several of her family members suffer from alcoholism or other substance abuse disorders.

She consulted me for enhanced support as she complained she was a "dry drunk", clinging onto "white-knuckle sobriety". She chronically felt irritable. Her hair test revealed a very low level of lithium in her hair, and I immediately started her on a low dose of lithium.

Six weeks after I prescribed nutritional lithium, Patricia came to my office in tears. She was partly joyful that she no longer felt a constant level of irritability, but she also realized with regret what it must have been like for her family to have tolerated her irritability and anger for such a long time. Low-dose lithium was able to transform her perspective on her life and improve her relationships with her loved ones.

## AMY

A 16-year-old patient, Amy, was diagnosed with bipolar disorder. On the medication Depakote, she was discharged from a psychiatric treatment center to a therapeutic school. She continued to experience angry outbursts and intense mood swings. There would be days where she would feel fine, while other days she would be extremely irritable and disruptive in class. She once articulated to me, "I can't control my outbursts—I need help."

Her nutritional laboratory tests revealed several deficiencies: most notably undetectable lithium. Although she was once on prescription lithium, she stopped due to the side effects. I recommended low-dose lithium at 10 mg per day, in combination with her Depakote. Her ability to control her mood swings and outbursts improved profoundly to the point that she was able to leave therapeutic school and return home to live with her family.

## PETER

A 4-year-old boy, Peter, struggled with severe symptoms of attention-deficit hyperactivity disorder (ADHD). Even at this young age, he was shunned by other children, and his parents were asked to remove him from preschool due to his disruptive behavior in the classroom. Desperate for relief, his parents tried different forms of "elimination diets", including the removal of dairy and wheat from Peter's diet, but failed to achieve any improvement in his behavior.

I learned that Peter had a strong family history of substance abuse, including alcoholism and cocaine addiction. When I observed Peter's aggressive behaviors first hand in my office, I ordered a Hair Tissue Mineral Analysis which revealed what I already suspected: non-detectable lithium. Not adding any medications, I prescribed 250 micrograms of lithium in liquid form to be taken once daily. Peter's annoying aggressiveness diminished and he was less hyperactive.

## GARY

Gary, a 35-year-old professional, sought help for chronic depression and "never feeling happy." He reported one episode of major depression where he required medications and had to take time off from law school. Gary recovered and returned to law school, got married, and had a successful career. He stopped antidepressants, as he reported inability to feel joy or sadness when taking them. Gary did not like the dulling of his emotions and feeling numb.

# Appendix

Gary grew up in a chaotic home where his father was verbally abusive and an alcoholic. He had an uncle who committed suicide. In addition to never "feeling happy," the most striking symptom that Gary's wife expressed concern about was his chronic irritability. Gary was easily frustrated and angry all of the time. He rarely had angry outbursts, but, as Gary explained, "sometimes I felt I was fighting hard not to explode." Gary's irritability was dramatically relieved with nutritional lithium. He reports that the change he experienced on 10 mg of lithium orotate was profound.

**For more case histories, please see www.LowDoseLithium.com.**

# Resources

For more information on low dose lithium and access to blogs and educational resources, please visit www.LowDoseLithium.com. This website offers information on a broad range of topics, including:

- Where lithium is found in the environment
- Growing uses of lithium in technology
- History of lithium as a dietary supplement and medication
- Latest scientific evidence supporting clinical applications of low dose lithium

## Other Books by the Author
*The Breakthrough Depression Solution: Mastering Your Mood with Nutrition, Diet, and Supplementation* (2016)
By James Greenblatt MD with Winnie To BS
ISBN-13: 978-1934716618

Despite the dozens of antidepressants on the market, millions of people who seek treatment for depression fail to find ongoing relief from their symptoms. Others must go through months of medication trials before finding the prescription(s) that works best for them.

The ideas as to what causes depression are not based on strong science, and our treatments are not working nearly as well as they should. Psychiatry

# Resources

is in crisis. The usual treatment method (typically based solely on a subjective psychiatric examination and construction of a symptom list) often leads to psychiatrists blindly searching for a medication that might work. Other factors such as nutrition, toxins, hormones, allergies, biochemical risks, and medical disorders are typically ignored.

No amount of changing this approach will work because the basic underlying concepts are wrong. Psychiatry needs an entirely new way of looking at patients. We must stop treating them according to lists of subjective symptoms, and we must stop acting as if one person were the same as the next. Instead, we must start seeing patients as individuals and then diagnose and treat their disorders accordingly.

In *The Breakthrough Depression Solution: Mastering Your Mood with Nutrition, Diet, and Supplementation*, Dr. Greenblatt uses what he's coined THE ZEEBrA approach to take readers beyond traditional treatment strategies toward healing. Dr. Greenblatt argues that, to treat depression, clinicians must understand the connection between mind and body and start looking at the unique biochemistry of each individual, including physical factors such as nutrition, genetics, hormones, and stress.

Based on decades of evidence-based research and over 25 years of clinical experience, the author discusses the latest technology and the many tests available to ensure that treatments are tailored to each individual for the best outcome possible. In this book, Dr. Greenblatt provides a personalized model of integrative medicine for mental health that can result in relief from depression and a renewed sense of emotional health. This groundbreaking book offers hope and treatment models that are proven, simple, safe, and effective.

*Integrative Therapies for Depression: Redefining Models for Assessment, Treatment and Prevention* (2015)
    Edited By James Greenblatt MD & Kelly Brogan MD
    ISBN-13: 9781498702294

# Nutritional Lithium: A Cinderella Story

*Integrative Therapies for Depression: Redefining Models for Assessment, Treatment and Prevention* summarizes emerging theories and research findings on various non-pharmaceutical therapies to treat mood disorders.

Supported by the review of nearly 3000 scientific studies, the book describes the concepts of inflammation, genetics, hormonal imbalance, gastrointestinal conditions, environmental stress, and nutritional deficiencies and their possible link to the pathogenesis of mood disorders. It also examines findings on various non-pharmaceutical therapies used to treat mood disorders including vitamins, botanicals, and other natural products as well as exercise, stress reduction, bright light, mind-body practices, and spiritual approaches.

With chapter contributions from over two dozen renowned physicians and researchers from across the country, this textbook is among the first of its kind to offer evidence-based approaches to integrative management of mood disorders in pregnant women, adolescents, and the elderly. Separating facts from fiction, the book provides practical information that clinicians can implement and share with their patients.

The book fills a significant gap in the conventional model of therapeutics for mood disorders. It is a valuable resource for psychiatrists, psychologists, family therapists, and all other clinicians who devote their days to caring for those afflicted with depression.


*Answers to Binge Eating: New Hope for Appetite Control* (2014)
By James Greenblatt MD with Virginia Ross-Taylor PhD
ISBN-13: 978-1461124122

Every year an estimated seventy-two million Americans diet, financing a weight-loss industry worth approximately fifty-five billion dollars. Despite the vast efforts put into weight loss, two-thirds of American adults remain either obese or overweight. Clearly dieting doesn't work, and failed attempts to lose weight encourage the development of disordered eating behavior.

# Resources

Many of those struggling with a disordered appetite compare it to being trapped on a roller-coaster ride. The feeling of the roller-coaster ride of restricting, bingeing, and chronic self-blame is never ending. There is the stretch of time when the car inches upward, when you feel a sense of progress. Then, without warning, you spiral downward in a great rush, having lost all sense of control. You crave, you eat, you binge. That momentary sense of calm and peace is once again shadowed by shame and guilt.

In *Answers to Binge Eating: New Hope for Appetite Control*, respected psychiatrist and eating disorder expert Dr. James Greenblatt explains how appetite is controlled by the brain's neurochemical systems, which rely on specific proteins for optimal functioning. The New Hope model described in this book combines the best in traditional and complementary approaches for recovery from appetite disturbances, food addiction, and binge eating.

While dieting providers a temporary fix, *Answers to Binge Eating: New Hope for Appetite Control* will offer a permanent solution based on scientific research to help you reclaim a healthy appetite with food. Following the New Hope model, you will find your answers to appetite control and get off the roller-coaster ride of food addiction.

*Answers to Anorexia: A Breakthrough Nutritional Treatment That Is Saving Lives*
**By James Greenblatt MD (2010)**
ISBN-13: 978-1934716076

This book offers the first new medical treatment plan in 50 years for anorexia nervosa, the "self-starvation" disease that affects adolescents and women of all ages in the U.S. and is now increasingly common in men. Based on cutting-edge research on nutritional deficiencies in anorexia that have been long ignored, the author explains how anorexia is a complex disorder with genetic, biological, psychological, and cultural contributing factors. In other words, anorexia is not primarily a psychiatric illness as has been believed for so long; rather, it is a medical illness of starvation that causes malnutrition in the body and the brain. Successful treatment must focus on correcting this malnutrition.

Dr. James Greenblatt has helped many patients with anorexia recover simply by correcting their nutritional deficiencies, and this book explains specifically which nutrients must be supplemented as part of treatment. *Answers to Anorexia: A Breakthrough Nutritional Treatment That Is Saving Lives* finally offers patients and their families new hope for successful treatment of this serious, frustrating, and enigmatic illness.

## Testing Laboratories
*Great Plains Laboratory*
   11813 W. 77th St.
   Lenexa, KS 66214
   Tel: 913-341-8949
   www.greatplainslaboratory.com

Great Plains Laboratory offers a broad range of nutritional and metabolic testing, such as the Metals Hair Test, which analyzes nutrients including lithium, iodine, zinc, copper, and potassium and toxic metal exposure such as mercury and lead.

*Trace Elements, Inc.*
   4501 Sunbelt Drive
   Addison, Texas 75001
   Tel: (800) 824-2314
   www.traceelements.com

Trace Elements specialize in hair tissue mineral analysis (HTMA) and provides levels and ratios for 36 elements, including lithium, zinc, copper, and magnesium.

Resources

## Nutritional Supplement Resources

*Pure Encapsulations, Inc.*
490 Boston Post Road
Sudbury, MA 01776
Tel: 800-753-2277
www.pureencapsulations.com

Pure Encapsulations was founded to formulate and manufacture the highest-quality line of hypoallergenic supplements available. Since its inception, the company has been the industry leader in manufacturing excellence and quality control, as well as a pioneer in the production of research-based and clinically relevant formulas. Sixteen clinical trials involving Pure Encapsulations products are currently in progress. These include studies at Stanford University, Michigan State University, and Mayo Clinic.

Available through health professionals, finished products are pure and hypoallergenic to optimize the long-term health of the most sensitive patients. An extensive product testing program involves verification of label claims, potency, and purity by third-party laboratories. Pure Encapsulations is NSF-GMP registered in the United States, is GMP certified in Canada, and exceeds the standards of the United States Pharmacopeia (USP) for supplement manufacturing.

*New Beginnings Nutritionals*
7797 Quivira Road
Lenexa, Kansas 66216
Tel: 877-575-2467
www.nbnus.net

New Beginnings Nutritionals provides high quality supplements specially designed for adults and children with special needs and allergies. Products are designed to provide support for special dietary needs, digestion, absorption, nutrient deficiencies, detoxification, immune dysfunction, and yeast and bacteria overgrowth.

*Radiant Life Company*
5277 Aero Drive
Santa Rosa, CA 95403
Tel: 888-593-9595
www.radiantlifecatalog.com

Radiant Life offers products and resources for optimal health and sustainable living. With an unyielding commitment to product quality and consistency, they strive to offer a highly curated collection of supplements that are whole foods based, ethically sourced, and which fit into the theme of ancestral nutrition and wellness. Whenever feasible, products remain free from pesticides, preservatives, GMOs, gluten and excipients of any kind. All foods and supplements have been prepared without solvents, high temps, bleaching, and deodorizers, and are packed both ecologically and safely.

## Physician Resources

*Green Medicine Online*
6839 Fort Dent Way Suite 134
Tukwila, WA. 98188
Tel: (206) 812-9988
www.greenmedicineonline.com

This website offers podcasts, articles, and information on nutritional medicine.

*Integrative Medicine for Mental Health: Referral Registry & Resources (IMMH)*
11813 W. 77th St.
Lenexa, KS 66214
Tel: 800-288-0383
www.integrativemedicineformentalhealth.com

IMMH provides referrals to and information on integrative medicine practitioners. The website also offers resources concerning integrative medicine and mental health treatment.

# Resources

*American Board of Integrative Holistic Medicine (ABIHM)*
5313 Colorado St.
Duluth, MN 55804
Tel: 218-525-5651
www.holisticboard.org
ABIHM is an association that establishes and promotes standards for integrative holistic medicine. It is also a resource for physicians desiring certification in integrative holistic medicine, as well as for those seeking physicians certified in holistic medicine.

*American College for Advancement in Medicine (ACAM)*
8001 Irvine Center Dr., Suite 825
Irvine, CA 92618
Tel: 800-532-3688
www.acam.org
ACAM is a nonprofit association dedicated to educating physicians and other health care professionals on the latest findings and emerging procedures in complementary, alternative, and integrative medicine.

*American Association of Naturopathic Physicians (AANP)*
818 18th Street, NW, Suite 250
Washington, DC 20006
Tel: 202-237-8150
www.naturopathic.org
The American Association of Naturopathic Physicians (AANP) is the national professional society representing licensed naturopathic physicians. AANP aims to increase awareness of and expand access to naturopathic physicians, help its members build successful medical practices, and expand the body of naturopathic medicine research.

*International College of Integrative Medicine (ICIM)*
P.O. Box 271
Bluffton, OH 45817
Tel: 866-464-5226
www.icimed.com

ICIM is a community of dedicated health care professionals advancing emergent innovative therapies in integrative and preventive health care. They conduct educational sessions, support research and publications, and cooperate with other professional and scientific organizations.

*American Academy of Environmental Medicine (AAEM)*
6505 E. Central Avenue, #296
Wichita, KS 67206
Tel: (316) 684-5500
www.aaemonline.org

The American Academy of Environmental Medicine is an international association of physicians and other professionals interested in the clinical aspects of humans and their environment. The Academy is interested in expanding the knowledge of interactions between human individuals and their environment, as these may be demonstrated to be reflected in their total health. The AAEM provides research and education in the recognition, treatment and prevention of illnesses induced by exposures to biological and chemical agents encountered in air, food and water.

Made in the USA
Middletown, DE
27 February 2025